R$1.00 A

DOCTOR HOMOLA'S
LIFE-EXTENDER
HEALTH GUIDE

Secrets That Help You Live Longer

DOCTOR HOMOLA'S LIFE-EXTENDER HEALTH GUIDE

Secrets That Help You Live Longer

SAMUEL HOMOLA, D.C.

Foreword by
JOSEPH L. KAPLOWE, M.D.

Parker Publishing Company, Inc.   West Nyack, N.Y.

Library of Congress Cataloging in Publication Data

Homola, Samuel.
    Doctor Homola's life-extender health guide.

    Includes index.
    1. Hygiene. 2. Longevity. I. Title.
II. Title: Life-extender health guide.
[DNLM: 1. Hygiene--Popular works. QT180 H768d]
RA776.5.H65   613   74-34098
ISBN 0-13-217240-2

To Martha with love

Books by Samuel Homola, D.C.

Bonesetting, Chiropractic, and Cultism
Backache: Home Treatment and Prevention
A Chiropractor's Treasury of Health Secrets
La Salud y Sus Secretos
Muscle Training for Athletes
Secrets of Naturally Youthful Health and Vitality
Doctor Homola's Natural Health Remedies
Doctor Homola's Life-Extender Health Guide

FOREWORD BY A
DOCTOR OF MEDICINE

This book *Doctor Homola's Life-Extender Health Guide,* might also be given the title "How to Help Yourself to a Longer and Healthier Life," for Dr. Homola explains in simple language how proper nutrition and other natural self-help methods, which are easy to follow, bring good health and prevent the premature aging so often found in those who should be enjoying a state of vibrant well-being.

No one wishes to grow old prematurely. In each heart there is always the desire to enjoy a long and useful life. To grow old prematurely and become afflicted with the disease of senescence results not only in becoming a burden to others, but also deprives the victim of the blessings that come with good health. Many diseases are the result of ignorance of the basic essentials necessary for attaining and maintaining good health.

By reading this book, you can acquire the knowledge you need to regain lost health and maintain good health. Guides to healthy living are clearly outlined on every page.

Dr. Homola has made a noteworthy contribution for those who wish to follow the path that leads to health, happiness, and a longer life, thus avoiding the needless suffering caused by premature aging. This book will relieve the suffering of millions of Americans who live miserably and die prematurely.

It is with deep sincerity that I recommend this latest book by Dr. Homola as a natural approach to better health and a longer life. Study this book and follow its recommendations, and your reward will be putting more years into your life and more life into your years.

Joseph L. Kaplowe, M.D.

WHAT THIS BOOK
CAN DO FOR YOU

In my practice as a chiropractor, I treat many middle-aged and elderly persons who complain of a variety of aches and pains. The primary concern of most of these patients, however, is longevity; that is, they are seeking some assurance that they will live a full, normal life.

I once told one of my 85-year-old patients that she would probably live to be a hundred, and I got a surprising reply: "I hope not," she said. "I don't believe that I could stand another 15 years of sickness and doctors' offices."

Needless to say, I was at a loss for words. For the first time, I realized that it's not enough to wish for a long life. *Life without health is not worth living.*

If you want to live a long, *healthy* life, you'll have to *plan* your life. You must adopt a program that aids nature in building a healthy body that functions efficiently. With the right program, you can relieve your aches and pains, improve your health, delay the aging process, and prolong your life. You can actually extend the vigorous, pain-free years of middle age, so that you won't look old or feel old until you reach your final days. Best of all, you'll be able to avoid frequent visits to doctors' offices.

No matter what your age might be, you should begin *now* to follow a program that teaches you how to live longer naturally. You don't have to allow the development of disease that results in a shorter or unbearable life. *Remember that the symp-*

toms of old age as we know it, and the common causes of death, are not a normal part of the aging process. With the program outlined in this book, you'll be able to prolong your life without suffering from the aging process. You'll be able to erase many of the outward signs of aging. Hundreds of home remedies are recommended for the care of ailments that cause suffering as well as premature aging.

If you're concerned about your health and you want to live your fully allotted life span without suffering from disease and premature aging, this book is for you. *Doctor Homola's Life Extender Health Guide* will provide the guidance you need to help yourself to better health and a longer life the natural way.

                                        Samuel Homola, D.C.

CONTENTS

LIFE-EXTENDER #6: How to Relieve Body Aches and Pains Quickly and Easily (cont.)

Cope with a Pain of Tic Douloureux • How to Speed Recovery from a Common Cold • How to Help Nature Heal Fractures • How to Handle a Hernia • How to Avoid Surgery for a Diaphragmatic Hernia • How to Remove Ear Wax • How to Control Psoriasis • How to Prevent Bed Sores • Dietary Supplements for Nervous Tremors

How to Improve Elimination by Correcting Constipation • Refined Carbohydrates Cause Diverticulitis and Colon Cancer • How to Cope with Rectocele • How to Relieve Gas Pains • How to Improve the Functions of Your Kidneys • Fasting: How to Lengthen Your Life by Restricting Your Diet • A Long-Range Diet for Longevity • Smoking Causes Premature Aging and Death • How to Sweat Out Poisons • Food Additives Can Clog Your System • How to Improve the Function of Your Liver

Digestion Begins with Chewing • How to Overcome Mild Allergy with Fermented Milk Products • How to Cope with Acute Diarrhea • How to Control Diverticulitis • How to Speed Healing of Stomach Ulcers • How to Cultivate Helpful Bacteria in Your Colon • Hints for Gall Bladder Sufferers • How to Handle an Irritable Colon

Stay Slim and Trim and Live Longer • Why Natural Foods are Superior to Refined Foods • Eat Five Small Meals Each Day • How Your Mind and Your Glands Can Affect Your Weight • Burn Excess Calories by Staying Active • How to Gain Weight Without Getting Fat • How to Delay Aging with Improved Body Mechanics • How to Lie Down and Straighten Your Spine

DOCTOR HOMOLA'S
LIFE-EXTENDER
HEALTH GUIDE

Secrets That Help You Live Longer

A Life-Extender Guide
for Better Health
and a Long Life

Very few people die of old age. With a life span of about 70 years, the average American is *killed* by *disease.* And in many cases, death is preceded by horrible suffering and disability. If you live properly and take good care of your body, you should live at least 125 years — without the suffering experienced by most "old" people.

There are a few places in the world where people live long, healthy lives. The Abkhasians of Russia and the Hunzas of India, for example, commonly live 100 years or longer. Many live to be 125 years of age. According to the May 9, 1973, issue of *Medical Tribune,* the oldest living Russian is 167 years of age. The oldest living American is 130. So a life span of 100 years — or even 125 years — is a reasonable and attainable goal.

In observing the life style of persons in countries where long life is the rule rather than the exception, it becomes apparent that living habits have a great deal to do with longevity.

A PROGRAM BASED ON
EXPERIENCE AND RESEARCH

After many years of practical experience, research, seven books, and more than 300 magazine articles in the field of health, I have formulated a health-building, life-extending program that I call "Doctor Homola's Life-Extender Health Guide." With ten simple "life extenders," you can improve your health, prolong your life, and effectively combat the development of ailments that are commonly associated with the aging process. My life extenders also employ natural remedies that can be used to provide immediate relief from aches and pains.

What could be more worthwhile than a self-help program that builds health, relieves aches and pains, and prolongs your life? Everything you learn in this book will do all this and more.

GOOD NUTRITION IS THE MOST
IMPORTANT SECRET OF LONGEVITY

My Life Extender #1 tells you how to select and prepare the foods your body needs to be truly healthy for a long life. Good nutrition is probably the single most important secret of good health and longevity. With a balanced diet of properly prepared *natural* foods, you can eat like a king and know that the food you eat will lengthen your life and make you feel better.

According to *Human Nutrition* (Report No. 2, 1971), published by the U.S. Department of Agriculture, "Most of the health problems underlying the leading causes of death in the United States could be modified by improvements in diet."

It's now well known that heart disease, the nation's No. 1 killer, is caused primarily by a bad diet. There is also some evidence to indicate that some forms of cancer may have a dietary origin. This means that you can extend your life by eating to *prevent* heart disease and cancer. When such information is available for the reading, you cannot afford to ignore it.

YOU CAN LOOK YOUNG
AS WELL AS FEEL YOUNG!

Life Extender #2 tells you how to take good care of your skin, hair, teeth, eyes, and other visible features that give your body a youthful, attractive appearance. And the methods you use to care for these features will keep them strong and healthy. The condition of your skin has much to do with your general health. So you'll want to give your skin as much attention as you give your teeth or your eyes.

Loss of teeth is a damaging blow to a youthful appearance. Worst of all, inability to chew food properly can result in a rapid decline in health. Since more teeth are lost to *gum disease* than to any other single cause, special care for your gums should make it possible for you to keep your teeth as long as you live — even if you live 125 years!

YOU CAN LENGTHEN YOUR LIFE
WITH THE PLEASURES OF SEX

There is now considerable evidence to indicate that a happy sex life is one of the secrets of longevity. Life Extender #3 will actually improve your sex life and make it possible for you to enjoy sex as long as you live. If your sex life is unsatisfactory because of bad health or misinformation, my instructions on "How to Increase Sexual Vigor" will prove to be a revelation.

NATURAL REMEDIES FOR
AGING ACHES AND PAINS

Many of the chronic ailments that commonly accompany the aging process can be prevented with Life Extender #4 and #7, which tell you how to improve circulation, flush wastes from your body, and stimulate your vital organs. You'll learn from Life Extender #8 how to improve your digestion so that your body can absorb the nutrients it needs to combat disease and the aging process.

When ailments and aches and pains do develop, Life Extenders #5 and #6 will provide you with the natural remedies you need to relieve your suffering safely and effectively. You can help yourself in the care of such ailments as constipation, arthritis, backache, headache, and insomnia — and in doing so, you can be assured of better health and a longer life.

A SPECIAL LIFE EXTENDER
FOR CONTROLLING BODYWEIGHT

If you're overweight, skinny, or physically unattractive, you'll be glad to know that one of my life extenders is devoted almost entirely to controlling your bodyweight and improving your physical appearance. The natural-foods diet I recommend, Life Extender #9, will fit right in with the type of diet you need to protect your heart and your arteries.

According to *Health Aspects of Aging,* published by the American Medical Association, atherosclerosis and obesity are two of the most common causes of rapid aging. So it's very important that you do all you can to keep your body lean and your arteries clean.

FOLLOW THROUGH
WITH AN ACTIVE LIFE

As you grow older, you should stay as active as possible in order to keep your heart healthy, your muscles toned, your bones strong, and your circulation efficient. It's also important to stay active simply to enjoy living.

If you put into practice what you learn from reading this book, you'll certainly improve your health and prolong your life. And just to make sure that you can take full advantage of all the extra years you'll gain by following my longevity program, you can use Life Extender #10 to keep your feet and legs strong and free from pain so that you won't have any trouble getting around.

HOW LUCILLE E. USED LIFE
EXTENDERS TO IMPROVE HER HEALTH
AND LOOK YEARS YOUNGER

Lucille E. was only 50 years of age when I first saw her in my office. She was already suffering from premature aging and chronic illness. She also suffered from constipation, arthritis, headaches, and a skin disorder of unknown origin. Her blood pressure was too high, and cholesterol was clogging her arteries, causing chest pain, leg ache, fatigue, mental confusion, and a variety of other symptoms. Lucille was pale and listless, and the premature gray hair that framed her unhappy wrinkled face made her look much older than she really was. Because of her chronic fatigue, she paid little attention to her dress and physical appearance. Her sex life had dropped to zero. In short, Lucille was being rapidly overtaken by an aging process that was being *speeded* by self neglect.

I instructed Lucille in self-help procedures that eliminated her constipation and relieved her arthritis. Home treatment for her neck arthritis literally banished her headaches. A change in her diet, with emphasis on the essential fatty acids, reduced her blood pressure and restored her skin to normal. The same diet opened her arteries and put an end to her chest and leg pains. Best of all, a renewed source of strength and energy permitted Lucille to once again concentrate on improving her physical appearance. She soon began to look youthful and radiant. For the first time in years, she had strong sexual desires. *By helping herself, Lucille started a chain reaction of physical improvement that apparently reversed the aging process.* She looked years younger and once again felt the verve of youth. Very likely, she also added 20 years to her life.

You can do as much for yourself as Lucille did. It's up to you. You can sit back and allow your health to deteriorate to the point where life becomes short and painful. Or you can help yourself feel better and live longer. Begin reading this book *now!* And put into practice what you learn immediately.

Summary

The life extenders outlined in this book combine a variety of self-help measures in an all-natural program that is designed to improve health, prolong life, prevent the common causes of death, and relieve the ailments that commonly accompany the aging process.

LIFE EXTENDER #1

How Certain Natural
Foods Can Help You
Roll Back the Years

Since good nutrition is foremost in building good health and extending your life, your first concern should be that of eating a variety of fresh, natural foods each day. Many of these foods should be eaten raw in order to assure an adequate supply of certain vitamins, minerals, and enzymes. Some foods must be cooked for easier digestion and absorption. How you cook a food, however, can be very important in preserving its nutritional value and its taste.

There are many concentrated food supplements that you can add to your diet to assure an increased supply of certain nutrients in special cases. As you grow older, for example, you may need additional calcium, phosphorus, and Vitamin D to keep your bones from getting soft or brittle. Bone meal is a good source of nutrients for aging bones.

You can decide for yourself which supplements you need most after reading this book. It's important, however, that you first have a good knowledge of the basic essentials of good nutrition.

HOW TO BALANCE YOUR DIET
WITH NATURAL FOODS

In order to get the essential nutrients in balanced amounts, you must eat some of *all* the basic foods each day. Nutritionists list four main classes of foods: (1) the milk group, (2) the meat group, (3) the vegetable and fruit group, and (4) the bread and cereal group.

For the variety you need for best health, you should divide the four classes of foods into *seven* groups and then make an effort to *eat at least one food from each group every day.*

Here are the recommended seven food groups: (1) leafy green and yellow vegetables, (2) citrus fruit, tomatoes, and raw cabbage, (3) potatoes and other vegetables and fruits, (4) milk, cheese, homemade ice cream, and other milk products, (5) meat, poultry, fish, eggs, dried peas, and beans, (6) whole grain bread, flour, and cereals. (7) butter and special unsaturated margarine.

Whenever you have a choice between a natural food and a processed or packaged food, you should always select the natural food. Foods that have been altered for packaging are not as nourishing as foods in the form supplied by nature.

Milk Products Supply Bone-Building Calcium

Since milk is man's best and most available source of calcium, every adult should try to drink two or more cups of milk daily. If you don't like milk, you can get your calcium from such milk products as unprocessed cheese, yogurt, and homemade ice cream. Remember that your bones and teeth are constantly rebuilding themselves. Without adequate dietary calcium, they will quickly deteriorate.

Persons who are allergic to the lactose in milk can usually eat or drink fermented milk products without any difficulty. The lactose in yogurt, cottage cheese, or cultured buttermilk, for example, has been converted to lactic acid by bacterial action.

One man who went on a "milk diet" to improve his health suffered a *decline* in health after several weeks of diarrhea caused by his allergy to lactose or milk sugar. When he switched to fermented milk products and a balanced diet, his digestive problems disappeared and his health improved immediately. There are many adults who do not have the intestinal enzyme they need to digest milk sugar.

If fermented milk products are not available to you and you feel that you need additional calcium, it might be a good idea to take bone meal and other natural supplements containing calcium. Remember, however, that your body cannot use calcium without phosphorus and Vitamin D. So make sure that any supplement you take supplies all three of these minerals.

You Need Protein to Build and Repair Muscles and Organs

Meat, chicken, and fish contain all the amino acids or protein building blocks your body needs to build tissue. Two or more servings of any one of them each day will help prevent the deterioration of aging. As you'll learn in other chapters of this book, there are good reasons why you should learn to prefer chicken and fish. You should eat seafood at least once a week for its mineral and iodine content.

Milk, milk products, eggs, and cheeses of all types are good sources of complete protein. Nuts, beans, and dried peas contain some protein, but with the exception of soybeans and wheat germ you cannot depend entirely upon vegetable or grain products for tissue-building protein. Vegetables and grains contain an *incomplete* protein that cannot be used alone to build tissue.

Persons who are knowledgeable about the amino acid content of the various vegetables and grains may be able to combine them to form a complete protein. There are good reasons, however, why you should *always* include some animal products in each meal. Vitamin B_{12}, for example, is found almost exclusively in foods of animal origin. And you need this important vitamin for building blood cells.

**You Need Fruits and Vegetables for Vitamins,
Minerals, Enzymes, and Carbohydrates**

In the vegetable and fruit group, you should eat at least one type of fresh fruit each day for Vitamin C and a couple of dark green or yellow vegetables for Vitamin A. As great a variety as possible, with at least four servings each day, would be best.

Vitamin C and Vitamin A strengthen tissue cells so that they won't fall apart so easily during the aging process. They also build resistance against infection and disease. Without adequate amounts of both of these vitamins, your flesh will sag and wrinkle and you'll be susceptible to all types of infections that threaten an aging body.

Fresh fruits and vegetables supply your body with a "clean" carbohydrate fuel for lasting, quick-acting energy. They also supply the indigestible cellulose fibers your bowels need to function normally. *Raw* fruits and vegetables supply important enzymes that you need to build youthful health. Cooking destroys enzymes in vegetables. So if a vegetable doesn't need to be cooked, don't cook it.

Whenever possible, begin your meal with a raw salad that contains a variety of cut vegetables. End the meal with a piece of fresh fruit.

Get Your Vitamin E from Whole Grain Products

When you purchase bread, always select the whole grain variety that has not been treated with preservatives. You can find such bread in the coolers of health food stores and in some grocery stores. If you want to make sure that your bread does not contain artificial additives, you can make your own bread with flour made from whole grains.

The cereals you eat should also be made from whole grains, and they should not contain chemical additives. In addition to containing preservatives, processed cereals are deficient in the roughage, Vitamin E, and other elements you need for good health and a long life. You need all the Vitamin E you can get from whole grain products if you want good circulation, a strong heart, and lasting sexual abilities.

Four or more servings daily of whole grain breads and cereals will probably supply adequate amounts of essential nutrients. If you feel that you need additional Vitamin E, see Life Extender #3 for information on how to take natural Vitamin E supplements.

Why Your Diet Should Always Contain Some Fat

We all know that too much fat in the diet causes overweight and hardened arteries. You must have a certain amount of fat in your diet, however, in order to absorb the fat-soluble vitamins. Fat also supplies certain fatty acids that are absolutely essential for good health. So while you must reduce the amount of fat in your diet, you should never eliminate it completely.

Vegetable oil is the best source of the essential fatty acids, and it is made up of the type of fat that won't harden your arteries. Some *soft* margarines contain a high percentage of essential fatty acids. When margarines have been completely hardened by a chemical process called hydrogenation, however, the essential fatty acids have been converted to a type of hard fat that is bad for your arteries. For this reason, you should avoid hard margarines, even if they are fortified. It would be better to eat natural butter than to eat hard margarines.

You should probably also avoid eating any product that contains "hydrogenated oil." Natural, unprocessed peanut butter, for example, contains a soft, unsaturated oil that won't harm your arteries. But when the oil has been hydrogenated it becomes a hard, saturated fat that is similar to lard or animal fat. Be sure to study the material on hardened arteries under Life Extender #4.

HOW TO COOK TO PRESERVE
YOUTH-BUILDING NUTRIENTS

In eating for better health and a longer life, it's not enough to select the right combinations of foods. If the foods aren't properly prepared, they'll lose many of their youth-building nutrients. Some foods may be eaten raw, and some must be cooked in a special way.

Fruits should always be eaten raw. And they should be washed before eating them unpeeled. Warm, soapy water may be needed to remove the oily film that accumulates on fruits and vegetables such as apples and tomatoes. Many germs can be found on produce that has been handled by picky shoppers.

If a fruit or vegetable has been waxed or sprayed with insecticide, it should be peeled before it's eaten or cooked. Unfortunately, apples, cucumbers, turnips, and other fresh foods are often waxed to preserve them and to give them a glossy coat.

A few vegetables yield nutrients best when they are cooked. It's great to eat raw carrots, for example, but you can get more carotene (Vitamin A) from a cooked carrot than from a raw carrot. Vegetables such as spinach and cauliflower are tastier and more easily digested when they are cooked. (Some *raw* beans may actually be toxic!) The trick in cooking any vegetable is to cook it just enough to soften the coarse cellulose fibers but not so much that you destroy the nutrients. When vegetables are cooked too long, in too much water, or with too much heat, many of the vitamins are lost or destroyed.

Steam Cooking Is Best

Cooking in steam or waterless cookware, just long enough to soften the vegetables, will preserve taste as well as conserve nutrients. You just put a few tablespoons of water into a special pot and then heat until the pot is filled with steam before dropping in the vegetables and putting on the lid.

You can purchase a special double pot for steaming vegetables, or you can make your own steamer. All you have to do is place a covered colander or a perforated pan over a pot of boiling water. The steam passing up through the vegetables will do all the cooking. Make sure that the vegetables are not submerged in the water.

Hints on How to Cook Vegetables

When you boil vegetables, always heat the water to the boiling point *before* dropping them into the water. And don't cut them until you're ready to cook them. Whenever possible, leave the skin on small vegetables and cook them whole. When you do have to cut a vegetable, cut it into pieces that are just large enough to permit cooking. Remember that the larger the cut sections of vegetables are, the greater the heat and the longer the time required for cooking. So while vegetables shouldn't be cut into small pieces they shouldn't be too large. It's never a good idea to shred a vegetable. The more of a vegetable that's exposed to air and water, the greater the loss of vitamins and minerals to oxidation and seepage.

When a vegetable is soft enough to penetrate with a fork, it is cooked enough. Don't ever cook a vegetable until it is mushy.

Some cooks add baking soda to cooking vegetables to preserve their color. This makes a pretty dish, but the alkaline soda destroys the acid Vitamin C.

Copper cooking pots are rare these days. But if one shows up in your kitchen, don't use it to cook vegetables. Copper destroys Vitamins B and C.

Always serve vegetables as soon after cooking as possible. Letting cooked vegetables sit exposed to air or steam results in a loss of vitamins. Leftover vegetables lose nutrients when they are reheated. Cook your vegetables fresh each day, and cook only as much as you can eat in a day.

Unlike vegetables that may be cooked by steaming, dry peas and beans *must* be boiled — in a new and special way. If you cook dried beans, for example, drop the beans into a pot of boiling water and cook them for two minutes. Remove the pot from the stove and let the beans soak in the cooking water for one hour before finishing the cooking. This method of cooking preserves nutrients by eliminating the customary 15 hours of cold-water soaking. It also permits you to use the soaking water as cooking water, thus retaining all the water-soluble vitamins and minerals.

When you do boil peas, beans, or some other vegetable in water, use the leftover water as soup, or simply drink it as "pot liquor." Water that has been used to boil vegetables is loaded with water-soluble vitamins and minerals. It's not a good idea, however, to drink greasy pot liquor. So don't add butter, oil, bacon grease, or margarine to cooking vegetables.

Make Canned Vegetables Your Third Choice

When you have a choice between fresh vegetables and canned vegetables, you should always select *fresh* vegetables. Your second choice should be frozen vegetables.

If you eat canned vegetables, don't throw away the liquid in the can. Instead, boil it down into a sauce and pour it over heated vegetables. About one-third of the water-soluble nutrients in canned vegetables are in the liquid!

Be sure, however, that you select canned products that do not contain monosodium glutamate and other artificial additives.

How to Prepare Frozen Vegetables

Always begin cooking frozen vegetables while they are still frozen. Just drop the vegetables into a pot of boiling water. This will prevent the loss of nutrients to oxidation and slow thawing.

Remember that vegetables that are thawed and refrozen not only lose nutrients but also become mushy and tasteless. When you shop for frozen vegetables, select packages that are not cracked or covered with ice. If a package shows evidence of thawing, don't buy it. The temperature of a freezer containing frozen foods should be maintained at zero degrees Fahrenheit.

Cook Your Meats and Eggs!

Meat should always be cooked before eating to make sure that it does not contain live parasites. There is just as much protein in cooked meat as in raw meat, and it's much safer to eat. So don't subscribe to any "health plan" that recommends the use of raw meat. Fish and poultry should also be cooked before eating.

It's usually best to broil meats over a slotted broiling pan so that they will be drained of excess fat and oil. No matter how you cook your meat, however, you should always cut away the visible fat *before* you begin cooking. Animal fat, in addition to contributing to overweight, tends to harden your arteries. So the less animal fat you have in your diet the better.

Boiling meats, like boiling vegetables, washes water-soluble vitamins and minerals into the cooking water. If you do boil meat and you want to use the leftover water as soup, it would be a good idea to first chill the stock in a refrigerator and then skim off the hard surface fat.

Contrary to popular opinion, it's not a good idea to eat raw eggs. Raw egg white contains avidin, a protein substance that destroys the B vitamin biotin. A raw egg may also contain disease germs if the hen is infected or if the egg shell has been cracked.

Try to cook your eggs just enough to harden the white without hardening the yolk. Cooking egg yolk until it is hard destroys the essential fatty acids in the yolk, which your body needs to keep the cholesterol in the yolk from hardening in your arteries. *Soft-boiled eggs are best.*

Beware of Cooking Oils

I usually advise my patients to avoid fried foods whenever possible. If you do fry something occasionally, you should use vegetable oil for "cooking grease." In addition to containing essential fatty acids that combat hardening of the arteries, vegetable oil has a higher smoking temperature. This means that it won't smoke or burn as easily as animal fat. When a fat or cooking oil begins to smoke, the fatty acids break down and form a substance that is irritating to the digestive tract. Each time a cooking fat or oil is used, its smoking temperature becomes lower. Some restaurants use the same oil over and over, until it smokes quite easily and becomes poisonous enough to cause diarrhea and other symptoms. This is one reason why you should never order fried foods in public eating places.

When you fry foods at home, always use *fresh* vegetable oil. Don't use the same cooking oil twice, and never use bacon grease.

Note: The polyunsaturated essential fatty acids of vegetable oils are best supplied by *unheated* vegetable oil. This is why I recommend adding pure cold-pressed vegetable oil to green salads.

According to some researchers, overheating vegetable oil may actually create a cancer-causing substance by breaking down the fatty acids. Most vegetable oils begin to break down if they are heated to 215 degrees centigrade for 15 minutes or longer.

FACTS ABOUT SPECIAL
ANTI-AGING FOOD SUPPLEMENTS

In other chapters of this book, you'll learn how to use vitamins, minerals, and other nutrients to speed the healing of various ailments. There are, however, some highly concentrated foods that everyone should include in his daily diet for health-building purposes. A good, balanced diet consisting of a variety of natural foods can be supplemented with delicious "wonder foods" that will contribute the additional nutrients you need to hold back the aging process. Even if you aren't concerned about growing old, these powerhouse food products will give you the verve you need to *feel* young. Many of these foods are so concentrated in nutrients that they are as potent as vitamin supplements. Try them all. Many of them can be added to regular meals or used as snacks.

HOW TO GROW
LIFE-GIVING SPROUTS

When seeds or beans sprout, they manufacture tremendous amounts of vitamins and other nutrients. A sprout is a "living food," capable of creating new life. It's delicious as well as nourishing.

There are many different types of seeds and beans that can be sprouted for food. Wheat seeds, alfalfa seeds, and soybeans, for example, are commonly used for sprouting. Your local health food store can supply you with untreated seeds that will not fail to sprout.

Alfalfa Sprouts

Alfalfa seeds yield a crisp, delicious sprout. To grow them, put about two tablespoons of seeds into a half-gallon large-mouthed jar. Tie a piece of old stocking over the mouth of the jar, or simply secure it with a rubber band. Rinse the seeds, drain the water, and then rotate the jar in a horizontal position so that the seeds will stick to the walls of the jar. This will allow proper ventilation. Let the jar rest on its side in a warm, dark place.

It's very important to rinse the seeds several times daily so that you wash away molds and bacteria.

The seeds should be fully sprouted in about three days. Further growth can be stopped by putting the jar of sprouts in a refrigerator.

Alfalfa sprouts are best eaten raw. They may be mixed in salads, soups, casseroles, vegetables, or placed in sandwiches. I frequently eat salads made up entirely of raw alfalfa sprouts. They are delicious with your favorite salad dressing.

Soybean Sprouts

Protein-rich soybeans probably make the most nourishing sprouts for combating the aging process.

First soak the beans overnight to facilitate sprouting. Use about four parts water to one part beans to allow for swelling of the beans. Then place the beans in a cloth-lined colander (perforated pan) and cover with a moist towel. Run cool faucet water through the beans several times a day to wash away molds and bacteria and to encourage sprouting. The more washing you do, the better.

After three or four days, the sprouts should be about two inches long. They may then be stored in a refrigerator until you're ready to cook them. If soybean sprouts are to be refrigerated or frozen for longer than seven days, however, they should be blanched or boiled for two minutes to destroy the enzymes that cause a loss of Vitamin C.

It's best to cook soybean sprouts so that you can eat the bean as well as the sprout. Just cook them long enough to remove the raw bean taste.

Whatever method you use to sprout seeds or beans, remember that there must be plenty of moisture with good drainage and ventilation. Sprouts will swell to about six times the original volume of the seeds or beans. So be sure to use a container that's large enough to hold the rapidly growing sprouts.

It's simply amazing to see a spoonful of seeds yield a jar full of sprouts. A sprout popping from a tiny seed is one of the wonders of nature. It's also one of our most inexpensive sources of concentrated nutrients.

Yogurt Improves Intestinal Health

Did you know that your intestinal tract is loaded with all kinds of bacteria? The colon itself serves as a home for certain types of bacteria, some friendly and some unfriendly. If the friendly bacteria are outnumbered by the unfriendly bacteria, you suffer from such common complaints as gas, constipation, and putrefaction.

One of the best ways to restore the normal bacterial content of the colon is to eat yogurt. Any of the common varieties of yogurt made from lactobacillus Bulgaricus, acidophilus, or Caucasicus bacteria will supply your intestinal tract with the lactic acid and the acid-producing bacteria you need to combat the growth of unfriendly bacteria. The acidophilus culture is most commonly used.

Yogurt also supplies acid that helps assimilate and absorb calcium, iron, and protein. It aids the intestinal bacteria in the production of Vitamin K and certain B vitamins. Some researchers maintain that yogurt is a natural antibiotic; that is, it destroys or hinders the development of disease-causing organisms in the intestinal tract. Yogurt used in enemas has been known to cure amoebic dysentery, which is a form of diarrhea caused by an intestinal parasite.

Although yogurt tends to kill unfriendly or disease-causing bacteria, it *helps* the growth of the bacteria that should normally be found in the intestinal tract. It's well known that various drugs and antibiotics taken orally will destroy helpful intestinal bacteria. The next time you are forced to take such drugs, be sure to eat a little yogurt to help replace and maintain the intestinal bacteria you need for good health.

If milk upsets your stomach because you are unable to digest lactose or milk sugar, remember that you can get all the nutritional benefits of milk from yogurt. Furthermore, the conversion of lactose to lactic acid in yogurt will actually *aid* digestion. Older persons who are deficient in stomach acid will especially benefit from eating yogurt.

To make sure that you get a good quality yogurt, you can make your own or purchase it ready-made in a health food store. Much of the yogurt found in grocery stores contains additives.

How to Make Yogurt at Home

All you have to do to make yogurt is to add a little acidophilus culture to whole or skim milk and then place it in a warm place for eight to 12 hours or until it thickens. (The cooler the temperature the longer it takes for yogurt to develop.)

You can speed the development of yogurt by placing small containers of milk and culture in a pan of water that's maintained at a temperature up to 110 degrees Fahrenheit. An electric frying pan may be useful for this purpose. I have used a closed box containing an electric bulb. If you purchase a commercial yogurt starter in a health food store, just follow the instructions on the package.

When yogurt is set or custard-like, place it in a refrigerator. If is is left out too long, it will become watery. Remember, however, that the longer yogurt stays in the refrigerator, the more acid it becomes. If you want a mild yogurt, don't make more than you can eat in a week's time.

Once you have a supply of yogurt on hand, you can make new yogurt by adding one tablespoonful of yogurt to a pint of milk. Eventually, however, you'll have to start over with a new or fresh culture.

If you haven't yet developed a taste for yogurt, try eating it with fresh fruit, sliced tomatoes, frozen orange juice, or chopped onions. When you do develop a taste for yogurt, you'll find it refreshing as well as tasty — and it will help build the intestinal health you need to live a long, *healthy* life.

**Double Your Energy
with Brewer's Yeast**

Of the 40 or 50 essential nutrients needed by the body, many of them are found in brewer's yeast. This includes practically all of the B vitamins, 16 amino acids (protein building blocks), and 18 minerals.

Brewer's yeast tablets can be purchased inexpensively at any drugstore or health food store.

Brewer's yeast *powder* is a lot more potent than the tablets. If you don't like the taste of yeast, however, you may have to take the tablets. Many people stir the powder into milk or juices. It can also be added to foods. I like to mix it in peanut butter, homemade bread, meat loaf, and soups. About four tablespoons of brewer's yeast powder daily should be enough.

The famous Tiger's Milk formula calls for brewer's yeast powder. Here's what an article in the *Ithaca Journal* had to say about the use of Tiger's Milk by a senior citizen's club: "The Senior Citizen's Club uses this recipe to relieve aches and pains. Chock full of vitamins, it can also be used as a pick-me-up. Tiger's milk cocktail: one quart of regular milk and one-half cup dried milk; one-half cup brewer's yeast, a small can of frozen orange juice (unsweetened). Keep refrigerated and use instead of aspirin."

You can, of course, flavor Tiger's Milk with any of the frozen fruit juices — or even ripe bananas. Just put all the ingredients into a blender and mix them thoroughly, preferably in skim milk.

Brewer's yeast will assure you of getting *all* of the B complex vitamins, so that they can work together in keeping your mind and your nervous system alert and healthy. A deficiency in any one of the B vitamins can lead to nervousness, fatigue, mental depression, and other symptoms. Yeast also contains ribonucleic acid, a substance found in the nucleus of every living cell. Some researchers believe that ribonucleic acid, or R.N.A., retards aging and improves memory.

Note: Be careful not to confuse baker's yeast with brewer's yeast. They are not the same. You should *not* eat raw, uncooked yeast cakes or dried baker's yeast. Yeast used to raise bread dough is made up of live yeast plants that will *rob* your body of B vitamins.

Combat Aging with Desiccated Liver

Like brewer's yeast, liver contains a wide variety of the nutrients that are known to be essential for good health and a long life. In addition to being rich in all the B vitamins, liver is a good source of blood-building iron and Vitamin B_{12}. A two-ounce serving of liver supplies more than six times the minimum daily requirement of Vitamin A, which you need for healthy skin and resistance against infection.

You should try to eat fresh liver at least once a week. If you don't like the taste of liver, you can take desiccated (dried) liver tablets with your meals. I frequently recommend both brewer's yeast *and* desiccated liver to my patients, since the liver contains Vitamin B_{12} and some unknown elements that are not found in yeast. Taken together, yeast and liver represent a potent food supplement that may give your body the boost it needs to overcome a variety of aging ailments. Desiccated liver is believed to contain an antifatigue factor that is especially effective for boosting the energy of senior citizens.

Sixty-year-old Emma B. came to me complaining of chronic fatigue and inability to think clearly. She also suffered from rheumatoid arthritis. "I've been to a number of other doctors," she admitted, "but none of them were able to help me. Other than my arthritis, they can't find anything wrong with me." I suggested to Emma that she try taking desiccated liver along with brewer's yeast, but only as a supplement to a balanced diet of fresh, natural foods. Six weeks later, she reported considerable improvement in her arthritis, and she no longer felt fatigued. "Maybe my trouble was all in my imagination," she said. "I don't see how dried liver and yeast tablets could improve my thinking." I assured Emma that the improvement in her health was not due to her imagination, and I advised her to continue taking the supplements.

Actually, liver and yeast supply such important vitamins as thiamine, niacin, pantothenic acid, pyridoxin, and other essential nutrients in *balanced* amounts sufficient to aid recovery from such chronic ailments as arthritis and nervous fatigue. Pantothenic acid and pyridoxin (Vitamin B_6), for example, may help arthritis by improving body metabolism, but they should be supplied with *all* the B vitamins. It's now well known that B vitamins work together. A deficiency in only one B vitamin can result in bad health, and an excessive amount of one B vitamin can create a deficiency in the other B vitamins. Dosing with Vitamin B_6, for example, increases the body's need for riboflavin, while dosing with riboflavin may produce a B_6 deficiency. So, rather than take only one vitamin in an artificial supplement, it may be better to take natural, concentrated foods, such as liver and yeast, to assure a balanced supply of *all* the vitamins you need.

Help Your Heart with Wheat Germ

Wheat germ is a powerhouse of energy-giving B vitamins and concentrated nutrients. It is also one of the few rich plant sources of complete protein. Wheat germ is best known for its Vitamin E, however, which is the vitamin you need for youthful blood vessels and a healthy heart. Most of the cereals and grain products we eat have been refined, eliminating the life-giving germ cells. (It is the germ of wheat that sprouts a new plant.) Without wheat germ, the average diet does not supply nearly enough Vitamin E for the best of health.

Toasted wheat germ, which can be purchased in any grocery store, makes a delicious cereal when eaten with milk and fresh fruit. Or you may simply add wheat germ to cereals, homemade bread, meat loaf, and other foods. It makes a delicious topping for homemade ice cream.

Once you open a jar of wheat germ, be sure to keep it in a refrigerator. And keep the lid on the jar. Exposed to air and warmth, wheat germ spoils quickly, developing a rancid flavor.

Build Strong Bones with Bone Meal

Two of the most common effects of "growing old" are brittle bones and loose teeth. Both are often the result of a calcium deficiency. Adequate calcium may not be absorbed because of a deficiency in stomach acid, or the diet may simply be deficient in calcium. (See Life Extender #8 for information on how to increase the amount of acid in your stomach for better absorption of calcium.)

Bone meal enriched with Vitamin D supplies all the elements your body needs to build strong bones. Two or more tablets with each meal will do wonders in strengthening weak bones and tightening loose teeth.

You can also take bone meal in powder form — stirred into soups or added to foods. I personally do not like the taste or odor of bone meal, so I take the tablets. I do, however, add bone meal to bread dough, meat loaf, and other foods that must be baked.

The older you become the more important it is to get adequate calcium, phosphorus, magnesium, Vitamin D, and other elements your body needs to build strong bones. You can get all these in their proper ratio from bone meal, a completely natural food made from finely ground beef bones.

In addition to strengthening bones, the calcium supplied by bone meal may have other beneficial effects. Muscle spasms, nervousness, insomnia, and other symptoms resulting from a calcium deficiency can be relieved by taking bone meal. One of my patients, for example, reported that her nightly leg cramps disappeared after taking bone meal to combat loss of bone around the roots of her teeth.

Many patients express concern about taking calcium or bone meal when they have "calcium spurs." Actually, such spurs form around joints that have been injured or irritated by arthritis and have nothing to do with the amount of calcium in the diet. In fact, such spurs will form even when there is a *deficiency* in dietary calcium. The body simply steals calcium from the bones in order to build-up a deposit around an inflamed joint. Taking calcium will *not* increase the size of such a deposit. So unless you have kidney stones or some other metabolic disorder that calls for a low-calcium diet, you can benefit from daily use of bone meal as a dietary supplement. (Available in meal or tablet form from health food stores.)

Seeds Contain the Germ of Life

Most seeds are concentrated sources of certain essential vitamins and minerals. In addition to providing phosphorus, iron, Vitamin B, Vitamin E, and protein, seeds also contain lecithin and unsaturated fat, both of which help combat hardening of the arteries. The high phosphorus content of seeds makes them valuable as a "brain food."

Remember, however, that seeds do not contain a complete protein. This means that seeds must be eaten with other foods if their protein is to be used in repairing muscles and organs. Also, the phosphorus in seeds must be balanced with calcium and Vitamin D supplied by other foods. An excessive amount of phosphorus supplied by an "all-seed diet," for example, can lead to excretion of calcium in the urine.

All types of peas, beans, brown rice, nuts, corn, wheat, and other kernels capable of sprouting new life may be classified as seeds. Sunflower seeds, pumpkin seeds, and sesame seeds, however, are probably the most concentrated in nutrients.

Sunflower Seeds Contain Sun Power

Sunflower seeds, which should be eaten raw, are packed with a variety of essential nutrients. One reason for this is that the sunflower is always facing the sun. As the sun moves through the sky, the sunflower actually turns its head so that it faces the sun every minute of the day. This keeps the seeds of the sunflower bathed in the life-giving rays of the sun.

You can grow your own sunflowers, or you can purchase the already shelled seeds in a health food store. A supply of seeds in your pocket or on your kitchen table will provide you with a handy and tasty treat as well as a nourishing food. In Russia, as in many foreign countries, sunflower seeds are a popular snack and may be purchased almost anywhere.

As nourishing as sunflower seeds may be, remember that you cannot live on seeds alone. I once read of a food faddist who died while trying to subsist only on sunflower seeds. A balanced diet is absolutely essential in building and maintaining health.

Pumpkin Seeds Boost Male Hormones

Pumpkin seeds are similar to other seeds in nutritional value — with one exception. Some researchers maintain that pumpkin seeds contain a hormone-like substance that improves the health of the prostate gland. They are also rich in zinc, which is found in large amounts in a healthy prostate gland. Just about every male over the age of forty has some prostate trouble, so it might be a good idea for every man to add pumpkin seeds to his diet.

Folk medicine in a number of foreign countries has long recognized the value of pumpkin seeds for prostate trouble. In an article by a German doctor, for example, we learn that "Only the plain people knew the open secret of pumpkin seeds, a secret which was handed down from father to son for countless generations without any ado. No matter whether it was the Hungarian gypsy, the mountain-dwelling Bulgarian, the Anatolian Turk, the Ukranian, or the Transylvanian German, they all knew that pumpkin seeds preserve the prostate gland and thereby, also preserve male potency. In these countries people eat pumpkin seeds the way they eat sunflower seeds in Russia — as an inexhaustible source of vigor offered by Nature."

Pumpkin seeds should be eaten *raw.* They're delicious alone or in combination with other foods. Try sprinkling a few of the seeds over your favorite dish.

Sesame Seeds Contain Calcium!

Most seeds are deficient in calcium, but not so with the sesame seeds. If you need additional calcium, try eating sesame seeds. Use them to flavor homemade bread, salads, sweets, vegetables, and other foods. Some people liquify sesame seeds in a blender and then use the delicious creamy liquid as a calcium-rich dressing or sauce.

Note: If you suffer from stomach ulcers, colitis, diverticulitis, or some other stomach or intestinal disorder, you may not be able to eat seeds unless they are reduced to a butter. Seeds trapped in inflamed intestinal pouches can trigger severe spasms or diarrhea.

Combat Hardened Arteries with Lecithin

As you'll learn with presentation of Life Extender #4, lecithin, which is rich in certain B vitamins and unsaturated fat, is a substance that helps prevent cholesterol from hardening in your arteries. It also helps form brain cells. If you eat raw seeds or cooked soybeans, you'll probably get all the lecithin you need to protect your arteries. You can, however, take a lecithin supplement made from soybeans. In granule form, it may be sprinkled over foods or stirred into juices. Two to four tablespoons daily should be adequate.

If you don't like the taste of lecithin, you can take it in tablet form. I personally prefer the tablets. Lecithin will, of course, be broken down into its basic components during the digestive process, but only to supply your body with all the elements it needs to manufacture its own lecithin.

Powdered Skim Milk Supplies Concentrated Protein and Calcium

We all know that milk is a good source of calcium and protein. When skim milk has been dried and concentrated in powdered form, it makes a concentrated food supplement that can be used to boost the food value of many other foods. It can be added to milk, bread, soups, custards, ice cream, and other foods that mix well with milk.

If you want a "high-protein drink," you can stir several spoons of powdered milk into a glass of milk. Remember, however, that many people are unable to digest milk sugar. If you suffer from intestinal gas or diarrhea after using powdered skim milk, don't use it again. Instead, use soured milk products.

Vegetable Oils Help Clean Arteries

Cold-pressed vegetable oil contains the polyunsaturated essential fatty acids we all need to counteract the hard fat in the animal products we eat. You should, of course, eat plenty of fresh vegetables and go easy on foods that contain animal fat. Everyone, however, can benefit from adding a couple tablespoons of vegetable oil daily to a fresh green salad. Safflower oil and corn oil contain the highest percent-age of essential fatty acids.

Seeds and nuts also supply unsaturated fat. If you're over-weight, however, you'll have to go easy on eating seeds and nuts if you take vegetable oil.

Note: Some researchers maintain that polyunsaturated fatty acids are easily oxidized in the body to form "free peroxy radicals" that damage cell membranes and *accelerate* aging. Vitamin E helps prevent this oxidation.

Actually, a couple tablespoons of unheated, cold-pressed vegetable oil daily should be enough to protect your arteries if your diet is properly balanced. If you take more, be sure to take a Vitamin E supplement. Too much vegetable oil, without adequate Vitamin E, may do more harm than good.

SPECIAL SUPPLEMENTS FOR SPECIAL CASES

Lucas B. never had paid much attention to what he ate. When his wife died, he ate very little other than packaged snacks made up of refined foods. He never bothered to eat fresh fruits and vegetables, and meat was so expensive that he rarely included it in his diet. Lucus didn't know it, but years of improper eating had already weakened his body and hardened his arteries. At 65 years of age, he could ill afford any additional neglect or abuse. His eating habits became progressively worse, however, and it wasn't long before he began to experience a variety of symptoms, includ-ing difficulty in thinking and remembering. A few years after the death of his wife, Lucus was placed in a nursing home where he deteriorated rapidly. He soon could not remember the names of his closest friends. Circulatory prob-lems began to develop in his feet and legs.

"He's just getting old," his family explained.

"Nothing can be done," his doctor emphasized.

Had it not been for a concerned friend, Lucus would have spent the rest of his life in a speedy, downhill slide toward total disability and death. With massive doses of B vitamins, especially niacinamide, along with lecithin, brewer's yeast, desiccated liver, and other basic food supplements, all supplied by his friend, Lucas regained his ability to think clearly. And in a short time, he returned home with fairly good health.

There are undoubtedly many elderly people who are suffering from nutritional deficiencies that are mistakenly assumed to be the result of the aging process. Anyone who does not take in an adequate supply of *all* the essential food elements, regardless of age, will be more susceptible to disease and disability. The older we become, however, the more we tend to neglect proper selection and preparation of foods. And since we *expect* our aging bodies to break down, most of us ignore what we consider to be symptoms of aging.

Numerous studies made of the effects of nutritional deficiencies on health and the aging process indicate that *good nutrition is probably the single most important factor in living a long and healthy life.* Yet, most senior citizens are *not* getting an adequate diet. A survey of almost 700 people over 65 years of age revealed that only one in 20 was eating properly. More than a third were not getting enough protein, more than half were not getting enough of Vitamins A and C, and more than three-fourths were not getting enough calcium!

If you have a good, balanced diet made-up of properly prepared natural foods (as recommended earlier in this chapter), you'll have all the basic elements you need for recovery and healing of your body in combating the aging process. It might be a good idea, however, to supplement your daily diet with some of the more important vitamins and minerals in order to withstand unexpected stress or illness. I usually recommend 25,000 units of Vitamin A; about 1,000 milligrams of Vitamin C; 600 units of Vitamin E; bone meal for calcium, phosphorus, magnesium, and Vitamin D; brewer's yeast and desiccated liver for the B vitamins; and a couple tablespoons of vegetable oil for the essential fatty acids.

Remember that it's usually best to take vitamins and other supplements in frequent small doses rather than in one large dose.

LIVE DIFFERENTLY TO LIVE LONGER

If you don't want to age prematurely and die of disease as the average person does, you'll have to live differently and eat differently. Remember that the average life span of 70 to 75 years is normal only for persons suffering from disease. Your goal in life should be to live 100 years or longer. This means that you must make a special effort to be *different*. And since bad nutrition is probably the major cause of premature aging and death, you must seek a good diet that includes concentrated foods.

Summary

1. A diet made up of a variety of all types of fresh, natural foods is the first essential for good health and a long life.
2. Fruits and vegetables should be eaten raw whenever possible. Eat something raw every day!
3. It's important that vegetables be cooked with as little heat and water as possible to preserve taste as well as nutrients.
4. Seeds and sprouts are packed with essential nutrients that delay the aging process.
5. Yogurt supplies acid-forming bacteria that help keep the intestinal tract healthy and free from disease.
6. A combination of brewer's yeast and desiccated liver is a potent formula for overcoming the fatigue and depression of old age.
7. Wheat germ, lecithin, and a couple tablespoons of cold-pressed vegetable oil daily will improve the health of your heart and your arteries.
8. The brittle bones of old age can be avoided or overcome with regular use of bone meal, milk products, and sesame seeds.
9. The zinc in sunflower seeds, and the hormone-like substance in pumpkin seeds, will help overcome the

prostate troubles of men who are over forty years of age.

10. Remember that the natural food supplements recommended in this chapter are *foods*. Proper use of such foods in conjunction with a balanced diet may make the difference between living an "average" life or living a long life.

LIFE EXTENDER #2

How to Renew
Your Look of Youth

Good nutrition will build your body *from the inside out,* so that you'll have the lasting health you need to live a long time. There are many *outward* signs of aging, however, that must be approached from the *outside* so that you will *look* young. How you care for your skin, hair, teeth, nails, and eyes, for example, will determine to a large extent whether you look young or old.

You may be perfectly healthy, but if your skin has been thickened and wrinkled by overexposure to the sun's rays, you'll look 20 years older than you really are. Oily skin or dry skin that is not cared for in a special way may become irritated, unsightly, or marred by blemishes. Hair that is dry, brittle, ridden with dandruff, or thin gives an aging appearance. Teeth that are stained, decayed, or missing will ruin the beauty of the most attractive body. No matter how healthy you may be, nails that "look bad" will give you a dirty or untidy appearance. Bloodshot eyes or baggy eyelids can be positively revolting. And so on.

With Life Extender #2, you'll learn how to care for the outside of your body. Remember, however, that health comes from within. It would be useless or futile to attend only to the outside of your body while ignoring the inside. Trying to hide signs of aging or neglect with make-up, clothing, colored glasses, nail polish, hair sprays, dentures, and other cosmetic appliances would not fool anyone for very long.

If you take good care of yourself *inside and out,* you'll glow with the health and vitality that combats the aging process.

HOW TO KEEP YOUR SKIN HEALTHY AND YOUTHFUL

In addition to adding to the beauty of the body, the skin has many essential functions. It registers pain, eliminates waste, controls body temperature, and wards off infections. It cannot carry out these functions, however, if it is not healthy. So, for your health's sake as well as for your appearance, your skin needs all the attention you can give it.

Sun Ages the Skin

Sunlight forms Vitamin D on the skin and has other healthful benefits. Too much sun, however, ages the skin and destroys the elastic tissue that keeps it tight and smooth. Warty brown spots, or "age spots," can also result from overexposure to the sun's rays. Continued overexposure may even result in skin cancer. So while it's important that you get out in the sun a little a couple of times each week, you shouldn't try to maintain a dark tan.

How to Soften Hard, Wrinkled Skin

Hard, wrinkled skin can be softened by soaking in oily water. Just fill your tub with warm faucet water and pour in a couple tablespoons of vegetable oil. Soak in the water for half an hour or longer. When you get out of the tub, pat off the excess water with paper towels and let your skin dry by evaporation. A thin film of oil remaining on your skin will hold in the moisture absorbed by your skin.

How to Cope with Age Spots

Once "age spots" form on the skin, there's not much that you can do about getting rid of them. Protection from over-exposure to the sun's rays will help prevent the spots from spreading. Some practitioners of folk medicine maintain that age spots can be lightened by rubbing them with cucumber juice or with sliced, raw cucumbers.

Ointments and lotions containing the B vitamin para amino-benzoic acid might help protect the skin from the aging effects of the sun. Vitamin B complex and Vitamin E taken orally might be helpful in preventing aging of the skin. You can get all the B vitamins you need from brewer's yeast and desic-cated liver, but it may be necessary to take supplements con-taining Vitamin E.

Note: When an "age spot" begins to develop a thick, crusty, or warty growth on the skin, a skin specialist should be con-sulted in order to rule out possible skin cancer.

HOW TO IMPROVE YOUR PHYSICAL APPEARANCE WITH YOUTH HORMONES

As you grow older, your muscles begin to shrink from in-activity. This leaves the skin loose and wrinkled. The best way to prevent this is to do simple barbell exercises. In ad-dition to maintaining muscular size, exercising with a bar-bell may actually help keep you youthful. There is now some evidence to indicate that there might be a connection be-tween lifting weights and the ability of the body to produce hormones (17-ketosteroids) that slow the aging process. In a controlled study of 75 men between the ages of 37 and 54, at the Veteran's Administration Hospital in Iowa City, Iowa, it was found that those who lifted weights showed an *increase* in the production of these hormones, while those who did not lift weights, but who exercised in other ways, showed a *decline* in hormone production.

You don't need to do a lot of exercises. Just stand erect and press a barbell from your shoulders to arm's length overhead.

Use a weight that's light enough to permit about eight fairly easy repetitions. You need only to exercise about twice weekly.

Note: The production of 17-ketosteroid hormones decreases during chronic illness, thus speeding the aging process. So it's important to stay healthy to be able to produce youth-building hormones.

How to Cope with Dry Skin

Dry skin is often inherited. It's also a common complaint among "old folks." It seems that late in life the skin tends to secrete less oil, so that the older you become the drier your skin becomes. If you find that soap and water causes your skin to burn and itch, you may have dry skin. This means that you'll have to observe special bathing procedures to keep your skin from becoming inflamed and cracked.

Actually, when the skin is not oily, it should not be washed very often with soap. In fact, skin that is so dry that it is scaly and irritated may have to be washed in plain water that contains a little vegetable oil. The use of soap may have to be limited to the face, hands, groin, and feet.

Oatmeal water is often used to clean irritated skin. You can buy oatmeal powder (at any drug store) to mix into your bath water. Or you can cook a little oatmeal, put it in a muslin bag, and then squeeze it in your bath water.

In the winter, when dry skin becomes worse, it may be necessary to rub olive oil into your skin after each bath.

A couple tablespoons of vegetable oil on a green salad each day may help soften and oil the skin from the inside. Vegetable oil contains Vitamin F, which is now known to be essential for good skin health. Without the essential fatty acids supplied by vegetable oil, the oil glands of the skin literally run dry.

Fish liver oil contains unsaturated fatty acids as well as the Vitamin A and iodine your body needs for healthy skin. It might be a good idea, therefore, to occasionally use a supplement containing cod liver oil.

Every winter, Claire E. suffered from burning, itching skin that frequently erupted in tiny red bumps on the back of her arms and on the front of her thighs. "My skin looks so bad sometimes," she complained, "that it scares off my boy friends."

Claire had inherited ichthyosis, or dry skin, that was made worse by winter dryness and the use of hot, soapy water. When she cut down on the use of hot water and soap and put vegetable oil in her bath water and on her green salads, her skin problems practically disappeared. "I don't have any trouble during the summer," she reported. "And I get along fine during the winter as long as I go easy on the soap and heavy on the oil."

How to Handle Oily Skin

The face and scalp are the oiliest portions of the body. For this reason, they have to be washed more often than the rest of the body. If you notice blackheads forming around your nose and forehead, it would be a good idea to steam your face occasionally with a hot wash cloth and then press out the plugs with a clean, soft fabric. This should be followed by a thorough washing with hot, soapy water. Allowing oil to accumulate in the pores of the face can result in unattractive spots and blemishes.

Don't ever try to clean your face with creams and oils. If your face is oily and the pores are clogged, only soap and water will effectively clean the skin. "Face creams" will only pack more oil into the pores.

A good rule to follow in cleaning oily skin is to wash it as often as necessary to keep it *dry*. Persons suffering from acne caused by oily skin may have to shower twice daily and then wash their face often enough to make it *peel* with dryness. Plenty of hot, soapy water should do the trick. It takes a strongly alkaline soap to cleanse oil from deep pores. Even then, it may be necessary to wash and rinse several times to open clogged pores.

Note: If your skin is normal, that is, if it isn't dry or oily, use a neutral or slightly alkaline soap and bathe just enough to clean the skin. Remember that excessive bathing of healthy skin will remove secretions that protect the skin from disease and infection.

Since the skin is normally acid, a fresh-water rinse containing a small amount of lemon juice or vinegar may be beneficial following a bath.

Home Remedies for Aging Skin Conditions

No matter what type of skin trouble you're having, there are some basic home remedies that you can use to ease your distress. These remedies are safe and effective and can be used by anyone.

What to Do About Sunburn

A cold bath, or cold, wet cloths will relieve the pain of a sunburn. It might help to add a little sodium bicarbonate to a tub of cool water and then soak in the water for awhile. Pat your skin dry when you get out of the water so that some of the sodium will remain on your skin.

Vinegar applied to the skin before blisters form may help prevent the development of a burn. Once blisters form, olive oil or a paste made from water and sodium bicarbonate might be soothing.

Prevention is the best treatment for sunburn. This means exposing your skin gradually to the sun's rays until you have acquired a light tan. This will give you the Vitamin D you need, and protect against the development of psoriasis and eczema. Because of the aging effects of the sun and the danger of sunburn, you should be careful not to stay out in the sun any longer than it takes to maintain the small amount of tan you have. When you reach the limit of your customary exposure, cover your body or get in the shade.

How to Ease Inflamed Skin

A cool, wet application, such as a wash cloth wrung out lightly in cold water, will relieve the discomfort of inflammation. Leave the application on until it begins to get warm and then change it. Continue to do this until the discomfort subsides.

How to Relieve Itching Skin

Corn starch or oatmeal that has been cooked will yield a starch that can be mixed in bath water for relief from itching skin.

To make a corn starch bath, mix one pound of corn starch with enough cold water to make a smooth paste. Then add hot water and boil the mixture until it becomes thick. Mix the paste in a tub of warm water and then soak in the water for 15 or 20 minutes. When you get out of the tub, pat your skin dry so that a thin film of starch will remain on your skin.

To make an oatmeal bath, boil three cups of oatmeal, put it in a cloth bag, and then squeeze it in your bath water. This will release oatmeal starch that can be mixed with the water.

Oatmeal water can be used to clean the skin when soap cannot be used. Use the bag of oatmeal as a washcloth after it has been squeezed in your bath water.

To make an alkaline bath, mix two tablespoons of baking soda into a tub of warm water. Soak in the water until the itching subsides.

A paste make up of sodium bicarbonate and water can be applied over small burns or itchy spots.

How to Smooth Rough Skin with a Corn Meal Rub

If your skin is rough, blemished, or pale, a corn meal rub will give it a soft, pink, smooth surface almost immediately.

Dorothy B. told me that she had not been in a bathing suit for years, and that she was horrified at the thought of swimming in public. "My skin is rough, blemished, and ghostly white," she complained. "I look like a stuccoed zombie, and I have a hot swimming date at the country club."

I told Dorothy to sit in a tub containing a few inches of water, wet her body, and then rub every inch of her skin with a little coarse corn meal the day before going swimming. Such rubbing, I explained, will rub away the outer layer of dead skin and stimulate the circulation of blood. If the rubbing is followed with a warm shower that's gradually turned down to cold, the result will be a smooth, pink skin that literally glows.

"I feel as if I have just shed a coat of paint," Dorothy said after trying a corn meal rub. "And my skin looks great!"

Rubbing your skin occasionally with ice cubes will help keep your skin bright and healthy by stimulating the circulation of blood. Simple massage will also improve the appearance of your skin. You should always use vegetable oil as a massage lubricant so that your skin can benefit from the Vitamin E and the essential fatty acids supplied by the oil.

(You can find many specific remedies for a great variety of skin conditions in my book *Doctor Homola's Natural Health Remedies,* published by Parker Publishing Company of West Nyack, New York.)

Feed Your Skin from Within

Good nutrition is essential for attractive skin. So many different vitamins and minerals are needed to build healthy skin that you must eat a varied diet to be assured of getting all of them. For nutritional insurance, however, and for special skin problems, it might be a good idea to take a few supplements. When there is a Vitamin A deficiency, the skin becomes dry, scaly, and easily infected. Skin diseases develop when the diet is deficient in Vitamin B. Vitamin C helps build the collagen that keeps the skin from sagging. The essential fatty acids supplied by vegetable oil help keep the skin soft and moist. And so on.

If you take vitamins in pill form, always select *natural* vitamins. In addition to containing vitamins we know we need, a natural vitamin supplement may contain unknown factors that are also essential for good health. It may be better to take *food* supplements rather than pills, however, in order to assure a *balanced* supply of essential nutrients. Fish liver oil for Vitamins A and D, brewer's yeast and desiccated liver for Vitamin B complex, and rose hip powder for Vitamin C, for example, can be added to a balanced diet.

Remember that you need protein and other nutrients to build healthy skin. Be sure to study Life Extender #1 for guidance in following a balanced diet.

HOW TO TAKE CARE
OF YOUR SCALP AND YOUR HAIR

The scalp is the oiliest portion of the body. If it's not washed often enough, an accumulation of oil, dirt, and dead skin may actually clog the pores of the scalp, shutting off the flow of oil. When this happens, there may be a tendency to refrain from washing the scalp, allowing the "dryness" to become worse. As a result, the scalp may actually become inflamed and cracked.

The case of Christine A. is a good example of what can happen when the scalp is not washed often enough. While applying physical therapy to the back of her neck, I noticed that her scalp was scaly and inflamed. I asked her if she washed her scalp every week. "Heavens, no," she replied. "My scalp is already so dry that it's cracked."

I explained to Christine that the scalp must be washed often to remove dead skin and to encourage the flow of scalp oil. I had a hard time convincing her, however, that she should shampoo her head a couple of times each week. When she finally did follow my instructions, her scalp healed and her dandruff disappeared.

If you can scratch your scalp with your fingernails and scrape up a scaly paste, your scalp needs washing. If you wait too long, your scalp will soon become "dry" and itchy. It's also very likely that you'll develop dandruff.

Try to wash your scalp at least once a week — preferably more often. If your hair seems to be too dry after washing your scalp, rub a little olive oil into your hair and then wipe away the excess oil with a dry towel. Your scalp will soon release all the oil your hair needs. A daily scalp massage will help distribute natural oil as well as guard against baldness.

How to Remove Hard-Water Minerals from Your Hair

When you use "hard water" to wash your hair, the minerals in the water combine with the soap and form a film that sticks to your hair. A vinegar or lemon rinse, followed by a fresh-water rinse, will wash away this film. Just put a little vinegar or lemon juice into a basin of fresh water and rinse your hair before stepping back under the shower.

A raw egg shampoo will remove hard-water deposits on hair. A vinegar or lemon rinse, however, is cleaner and not so messy.

Rainwater is "soft water," and does not contain minerals that will stick to hair. If soft water is not available in your home, and you don't want to bother with rinses to remove mineral deposits, try using a little rainwater.

How to Prevent Baldness

Baldness is primarily a problem of men. An increasing number of women, however, are becoming bald. This may be due to excessive use of hair sprays, rinses, dyes, and other unnatural chemicals on the hair. I suspect that use of wigs and hair pieces will contribute even more to female baldness in the years to come. It's well known that the scalp should be brushed and massaged to stimulate the circulation of blood to the hair roots. Women who use wigs daily may literally suffocate the scalp by shutting out sunlight and air and by reducing the flow of blood to hair roots. Once the scalp becomes thin and tight from neglect, the hair simply dies from lack of attention and nutrients.

Always massage your scalp when you wash your hair. Go bareheaded as often as possible. Concentrate on keeping the muscles of your forehead relaxed. A tense and wrinkled brow interferes with the blood flow to hair roots by tightening scalp muscles. Lying on a slant board will increase the flow of blood to your scalp.

All of the B vitamins are important in keeping a healthy head of hair. One nutritionist singles out inositol (one of the B vitamins) as essential in preventing baldness. (Sunflower seeds are a good source of inositol.) The two best sources of *all* the B vitamins are brewer's yeast and desiccated liver. Remember that B vitamins are most effective when they all work together. Some people have reported *new growth of hair and restoration of color* after prolonged use of both yeast and liver tablets.

Male Pattern Baldness

Unfortunately for some men, the male sex hormones can contribute to "male pattern baldness" that starts early in life. The only sure way to avoid such baldness is to undergo castration — a procedure no man would undergo just to keep the hair on his head. So if you become bald in spite of everything you do to save your hair, blame it on your hormones.

More About Gray Hair

Gray hair can be beautiful. If you are fairly young, however, and you are graying prematurely, you might be able to prevent excessive graying with nutritional supplements. Pantothenic acid, para aminobenzoic acid, and folic acid, which are B vitamins found in wheat germ, liver, and brewer's yeast, are believed to be helpful in restoring color to graying hair.

HOW TO COPE WITH BODY ODORS

Most of us are so conscious of body odors that we use a variety of commercial preparations to mask odors that seem to develop no matter how often we bathe. Actually, what most of us consider to be offensive odors are, for the most part, normal and natural. In fact, at one time, body odors were so acceptable that they were thought to be sexually stimulating. It was Charles Baudelaire, a 19th century French poet, who telegraphed his mistress: "Don't wash. I'm coming home tomorrow." Today, the trend is to eliminate all body odors.

The most offensive odors come from the apocrine glands that are located under the arms and in the groin area. Bacteria feeding upon the secretions of these glands, where there is little or no circulation of air, produce most of the odor.

If you're bothered with body odors and you're unable to take a daily bath for some reason, you should at least wash your feet, groin, and underarms with a washcloth. Don't try to stop these odors with antiperspirants. Such preparations clog the apocrine glands and may lead to the development of boils, cysts, or tumors.

As you grow older, the apocrine glands, which are associated with sexual glands, become less active and therefore cause less odor. This is one reason why many older people tend to bathe less. They simply do not develop the body odors they once had.

FINGERNAILS REFLECT
HEALTH AND LIVING HABITS

Like your skin, your nails can reflect poor health and nutritional deficiencies. Iodine or protein deficiency, for example, can result in brittle nails. (Seafood supplies protein as well as iodine. Gelatin will often restore strength to brittle nails. Remember, however, that gelatin is not a complete protein and cannot be used alone to build tissue.)

The size, shape, and color of the nails are often helpful in the diagnosis of disease. Pale nails, for example, may be a sign of anemia. Nails that are concave like spoons are often associated with severe, chronic anemia. Blue nails may result from an oxygen deficiency caused by a heart or circulatory disorder. In certain types of lung disease, the nails may be rounded like a watch crystal. Tiny spots or hemorrhages may appear under the nails if there is inflammation of the lining of the heart. And so on. If your nails appear to be abnormal, be sure to show them to your doctor.

Keep your nails clean! Dirt under the edges of your nails reflects unfavorably upon your personal habits. Don't scrape under your nails with sharp metallic objects. Scratched nails catch dirt that is difficult to remove. Use wooden or plastic strips to clean under the edges of your nails.

TAKE A LOOK AT YOUR EYES

When you see someone with bloodshot eyes, baggy eyelids, or dark circles around their eyes, your first thought may be that the individual looks unhealthy, tired, or old. Nutritional deficiencies that affect the appearance of the eyes can certainly contribute to premature aging. When the eyeballs are dry and inflamed from a Vitamin A deficiency, for example, you can be sure that the tissue cells of the body are not strong enough to resist invasion by germs. Bluish eyeballs caused by anemia or iron deficiency means that there is an oxygen deficiency in the body. Baggy eyelids may point to kidney disease or heart trouble that allows water to accumulate in the tissues. Swollen eyes may result from allergic reactions. Dark, circled eyes may mean that nutritional deficiency or emotional stress is depriving the body of the sleep it needs to recover from fatigue and stress.

Arcus senilis. When the iris or colored portion of the eye is circled with a white ring, it may be a sign of an excessive amount of heart-damaging cholesterol in the blood. (Yellowish-white deposits may also build-up in the eyelids.)

Practically any abnormality of the eyes reflects stress, deficiencies, and other factors that can speed the aging process.

How to Make Eye Wash
for Dry, Scratchy Eyes

As we grow older, the tear ducts of our eyes tend to "dry out," leaving the e_'eballs dry and inflamed. Your doctor can recommend special eye drops for temporary relief.

You can make an eye-wash solution at home by following this simple formula: Take a moderately-heaped teaspoonful *each* of bicarbonate of soda, borax, and table salt and dissolve them into a quart of boiled water. Add a tablespoonful of glycerine. The glycerine will provide the oil your eyeballs need for lubrication. Filter the solution before using it on your eyes. It might also be a good idea to soak a piece of cotton in the solution and wipe your eyelashes before attempting to wash out your eyes.

A simple eye rinse. You can make a simple eye rinse for tired, dust-clogged eyes by following this formula: Let a pint of water stand overnight so that all the chlorine in the water can escape as gas. Then add a level teaspoonful of table salt. Make sure that all the salt dissolves into the water and that there is no dust in the bottle. You can drop the solution into your eyes with an eyedropper, or you can wash cach eye with an eye cup.

Eyelashes and Chronic Eye Inflammation

When your eyeballs are so scratchy and inflamed that it feels as if you have sandpaper under your eyelids, a cold washcloth over your eyes will provide soothing relief. If a scratchy irritation persists, you may have an eyelash that has turned in against your eyeball. An ophthalmologist can provide relief by removing the hair.

Vitamin A and Night Blindness

If you have trouble seeing at night, don't just assume that it's due to the aging process. It might be night blindness caused by a Vitamin A deficiency. Take several thousand units of Vitamin A daily for a few weeks. If that doesn't help, see your doctor. Remember that taking excessive amounts of Vitamin A over a long period of time may have harmful side effects.

Diabetes Can Affect Vision

Poor vision during the day may mean diabetes. Be sure to have your blood sugar checked if your vision becomes bad for no apparent reason. Yellowish-orange deposits can sometimes be seen in the eyelids of diabetic patients.

Symptoms of Glaucoma and Cataract

If your field of vision seems to be reduced, or if you see rainbows or halos around electric lights, your eyes should be checked for cataracts and glaucoma. Persons with cataracts can often see better at night than in the daytime. The reason for this is that in the daytime the pupil becomes smaller in response to sunlight, reducing the opening that allows you to see around small cataracts.

Senile cataracts are common after 50 years of age, and often begin at about age 40.

Using Your Eyes to Detect Disease

Like your fingernails, sudden or abnormal changes in the appearance of your eyes may point to the presence of disease in your body. Eyes that bulge excessively, for example, may mean hyperthyroidism or disease of the thyroid gland. Eyes that are sunken because of deterioration of the fatty pads behind the eyes may have a special meaning.

When an eyelid droops for no apparent reason, your doctor should examine your chest for signs of tumors or bony growths that may be pressing against important nerve centers.

When one pupil is larger than the other, have an opthalmologist and a neurologist examine your eyes and your nervous system. Glaucoma, for example, can create enough pressure in an eyeball to enlarge the pupil. A neck rib, a brain tumor, or some other abnormality can dilate a pupil by putting pressure on some part of the nervous system. The neck rib may be harmless, but the tumor may be deadly.

If you have to have your glasses changed more often than once every two years, see an optometrist or an opthalmologist for an eye examination. Be checked specifically for glaucoma.

Presbyopia: Old Age Vision

Most people over the age of forty can see better with glasses. One reason for this is that the lens of the eye loses the elasticity it needs to respond to the pull of tiny muscles that focus the lens. Don't be ashamed to wear glasses if you need them. People who brag that they can see great distances without the aid of glasses often need glasses for reading and other close work.

Many people who were once nearsighted find that they can see better at a distance after the age of 43 or so. This is the result of a change in the lens or the eye muscles, and may actually *reverse* the sight problems they once had. Doctors term this change "presbyopia."

How many times have you seen a middle-aged or elderly person hold a book or newspaper at arm's length in order to read the print? You don't have to let that happen to you. Be sure to have your eyes examined — and your glasses changed — if your vision seems to be changing.

Self Help for Eye Discomfort

How to use a hot compress. For relief of pain in infections around the eye, a hot, moist compress might be helpful. Wring out a piece of flannel in 115 degrees water (or as hot as can be withstood) and place it over the closed eye. Renew the compress every minute for 10 or 15 minutes several times a day.

If the pain seems to get worse after applying heat, try using a cold pack.

How to use a cold compress. Cold compresses are usually best for relieving inflammation of the eye. Fold a piece of cotton cloth four or five times to make a pad about 1½ inches square. Wet the pad and lay it on a block of ice before placing it on the closed eye. Change the pad when it becomes warm.

How to massage the eyeball. The eyeball is filled with a fluid that is constantly filling and draining. You can stimulate the circulation of this fluid by massaging the eyeball.

Press a finger against the closed upper eyelid. Press just hard enough to indent the eyeball slightly, but not enough to cause pain. Press about 20 times, three times a day.

Eyeball massage might help relieve the symptoms of glaucoma by forcing drainage of fluid from the eye. Talk to your doctor, however, before using the massage.

Large doses of Vitamin C, many times larger than the recommended daily requirement, have reportedly been useful in the treatment of glaucoma. (See *New Hope for Incurable Diseases,* by E. Cheraskin, M.D., Arco Publishing Company, New York.)

HOW TO KEEP YOUR
TEETH FOR A LIFETIME

If you still have all your teeth when you reach 40 years of age, you have probably taken pretty good care of your teeth. *After* the age of forty, however, the condition of your *gums* may determine how much longer you keep your teeth. It's well-known that the gums begin to recede after the age of 30. If special gum-cleaning procedures aren't used, infection can lead to loss of teeth from pyorrhea or periodontal disease. This dreaded disease accounts for more lost teeth than all other factors combined. Three out of every four Americans, and almost 100 percent of all Americans over the age of 65, have periodontal disease. So it's unlikely that you'll be able to escape the disease completely. You can prevent loss of teeth, however, by carrying out certain simple procedures at home.

Always Clean Your Teeth After Eating

Brush your teeth after each meal. Use a *soft* brush and make sure that the bristles slip up under the edges of your gums. Use short back-and-forth strokes with the tooth brush angled toward the gum margin. If deposits aren't removed from under the edges of the gums at least once every 24 hours, they form a sticky plaque that feeds bacterial infection. This can lead to the formation of gum pockets and bone loss around the roots of perfectly healthy teeth.

Use Dental Floss Regularly

Just to make sure that no tartar or plaque forms under the gum margins between your teeth, you should clean your teeth with dental floss at least once each day, preferably before retiring at night. Slip the floss up and down *each side of each tooth* several times, moving the floss as far under the edge of the gum as you can. *Unwaxed* dental floss will do a better job of raking deposits off your teeth.

Have Your Teeth Scaled Periodically

No matter how good a job you do cleaning your teeth and your gums, you should see your dentist occasionally so that he can scrape away deposits in hard-to-get-to spots. It may even be necessary to deaden your gums with an anesthetic in order to permit scaling deep beneath the gum margins.

If your gums bleed during brushing, or if you have bad breath in spite of regular cleaning, you may already have deep pockets around the roots of your teeth. If these pockets aren't removed surgically by a dentist or a periodontist, bacterial activity in the pockets may actually eat away the bone that supports the roots of your teeth.

Note: Loose teeth almost always mean periodontal disease. A blue line on gum margins around natural teeth is a symptom of lead poisoning.

How to Wash Out Gum Pockets

Once pockets form under the edges of the gums, cleaning becomes more difficult. Even gum surgery sometimes fails to eliminate all the pockets. So it's a good idea for everyone to use an oral irrigation appliance to wash out pockets and

crevices under the edges of the gums. (Even healthy gums
have a tiny crevice under the gum margins. When the gums
recede, however, or become diseased, these crevices deepen
to form pockets.)

An oral irrigation appliance, sold in drug stores, generates
a tiny, forceful stream of water than can be directed under
the gum margins. You'll be surprised at the "garbage" you
can wash out from under the edges of your gums after you
have brushed your teeth.

Increase Your Intake of
Calcium to Protect Your Teeth

There is now some evidence to indicate that bone loss
around the roots of the teeth may be one of the first signs
of calcium deficiency. Just to make sure that your body has
the raw materials it needs to build bone, you should take
bone meal tablets regularly. A little sunshine and skim milk
daily might also be helpful.

Vitamin C will help strengthen gum tissue, and Vitamin A
will help your gums resist infection.

Strengthen Your Teeth by
Eating Raw Fruits and Vegetables

You can strengthen your teeth and stimulate bone formation around the roots of your teeth by eating raw fruits and
vegetables, such as apples, carrots, celery, and raw sweet
potatoes. Yellow fruits and vegetables contain Vitamin A
(carotene) as well as Vitamin C.

Persons who eat nothing but cooked and refined foods
may actually lose calcium in their jaw bones from lack of
adequate chewing exercise. Raw fruits and vegetables afford
ideal exercise for the teeth, and they provide essential nutrients for your gums.

When you are unable to brush your teeth after eating,
finish your meal with a piece of raw fruit and then rinse your
mouth thoroughly with water. Squish the water between your
teeth to wash away lodged food particles.

How to Use Interdental Stimulators

Interdental stimulators made from balsa wood will stimulate the gums as well as clean the teeth. These small sticks of soft wood are simply pressed between the teeth and against the gum margin in much the same way you'd use a toothpick. You can purchase interdental stimulators in matchbox-size packages that you can carry around in your purse or your pocket. Take some with you when you "eat out" or go on picnics. Use them whenever it's not possible to brush your teeth.

Don't Clench Your Teeth

When your gums become diseased and your teeth loosen, you may develop a tendency to clench your teeth. Don't do it! Such clenching can *speed* the development of periodontal disease, and it can loosen *healthy* teeth by damaging the membranes that hold them in their bony sockets.

If you feel that your teeth do not fit together properly, have a dentist check your teeth for malocclusion. It might be that all he needs to do to correct your bite is to grind down a couple of teeth that have drifted out of alignment. Remember that when a tooth is extracted and is not replaced by a bridge, it's not uncommon for the rest of the teeth to "drift" or move toward the empty space. This can lead to malocclusion, which can contribute to the development of periodontal disease. Try to avoid losing a tooth whenever possible. If a tooth must be extracted, have it replaced with a denture as soon as possible.

Diabetes Can Make Gum Disease Worse

If gum troubles persist in spite of the cleaning procedures you use, ask your doctor for a blood sugar test. Gum infections are difficult or impossible to control when they are complicated by diabetes. Bacteria in gum pockets thrive on sugar-rich blood.

Summary

1. Good health must be built from the inside, but the outward appearance of your skin, hair, nails, and

teeth will have a lot to do with how youthful you look.

2. In many cases, the skin becomes drier as the body becomes older. Dry skin requires less use of soap and more use of oil.

3. Dandruff and "dry scalp" are often caused by failure to wash the head often enough to remove oil and dead skin caked on the scalp.

4. Growth of hair can be aided by massaging your scalp and increasing your intake of B vitamins.

5. A plus for the aging process: body odors become *less* of a problem with decreased function of the apocrine sweat glands.

6. Abnormal fingernails often reflect the presence of disease or deficiency in the body.

7. A drooping eyelid, an uneven pupil, a white ring in the iris of the eye, and other changes in the eyes should be brought to the attention of a physician.

8. If you see halos around electric lights, see better at night than in the daytime, or have to have your glasses changed more often than once every two years, your eyes should be checked for cataracts and glaucoma.

9. Bleeding gums, bad breath, or loose teeth may mean periodontal disease that could lead to loss of teeth if not corrected immediately.

10. The teeth and the gum margins should be cleaned regularly with a toothbrush, dental floss, and an oral irrigation device — in addition to regular visits to a dentist.

LIFE EXTENDER #3

How to
Increase Sexual Vigor

"Age alone does not make a man impotent, and age alone does not erase desire from the female."

This statement from a recent issue of a popular health magazine reflects a new trend of thought that now *encourages* the pursuit of sexual satisfaction by "old people." There is, in fact, evidence to indicate that *most people can enjoy sexual activities at least into their eighties.* Many sexually inactive people under the age of 80 simply suppress their sexual desires because of taboos and misinformation. Some are embarrassed to admit that they still have strong sexual desires.

According to Kinsey's studies back in 1948 (*Sexual Behavior in the Human Male*), nearly 30 percent of males over the age of 70 were inactive sexually. Many of these were undoubtedly suppressing their desires in conforming with prevailing customs. Some were truly impotent. Whether you are a male or female, you should do everything you can to encourage your sexual desires and to stay active sexually. No matter how old you may be, *if you feel a desire to continue regular sexual activity you should do so.*

Kinsey told of one 70 year old white male who averaged seven sexual climaxes a week, and of an 88 year old Negro male who was still having intercourse with his 90 year old wife as often as once a week. The May 9, 1973, issue of *Medical Tribune* published the story of a 90 year old Mexican whose 31st bride was only 25 years of age!

You might be among those who will be able to enjoy the pleasures of sex late in life. In this day of sexual enlightenment, you don't have to be inhibited by ignorance or puritanical standards. Don't suppress your desires and feelings and lock yourself away as a worn-out relic because of your age. Remember that pursuit of sexual pleasure maintains sexual capacity. In the case of sex, it's certainly true that *if you don't use it you'll lose it.*

PRACTICE MAKES PERFECT

Research now indicates that the younger a person begins an active sex life, and the more often he satisfies his sexual desires, the longer he keeps his sexual powers. In other words, the more sexual activity you have the more capable you are — much like the aged athlete who maintains his ability to jog several miles by jogging a couple of times each week. Like the muscles of your body, your sexual organs are strengthened by regular use.

A 65 year old man who was contemplating a second marriage expressed concern to me about losing his "manhood." He had been divorced for several years and was going with a 50 year old woman. "I want to marry her," he confided, "but I'm wondering if I have enough shots left in me for another marriage." I assured the man that no one had a predetermined number of "shots" that could be used up. "In fact," I said, "the more active you have been over the years the better your chances of continuing an active sex life."

Of course, as you grow older, you may not be able to indulge in sexual activity as often as you did when you were younger. And it may take a little longer to get ready and to complete the act. But quality can replace quantity. You may even enjoy sexual love *more* as you grow older, even if it comes only occasionally. The thing to remember is that you should *encourage* your sexual feelings. Just be guided by the way you feel. You don't have to abandon the pleasures of sex just because "most people" your age are no longer active sexually. Besides, the notion that "old people" are not interested in sex is largely a myth. If you suppress your own desires because of statistics and opinions, you are depriving yourself unnecessarily. As a result, you will eventually lose your ability to perform sexually.

Even if you can't bring yourself to pursue sex for the pleasure it offers, there are other good reasons why you should stay sexually active if you are able to do so.

SEX IMPROVES HEALTH
AND PROLONGS LIFE

There is now some evidence to indicate that sexual activity delays the aging process. It's also good exercise! In addition to the actual muscular effort required to perform sexual intercourse, a sexual climax has a stimulating effect on the heart, lungs, and blood circulation. The entire nervous system is jolted, aiding in the production of hormones. Sexual excitement has been known to relieve such chronic disorders as hay fever and sinus congestion. There is no drug, nor any exercise, that offers the combined effects of pleasure and stimulation in so beneficial a manner.

So even if you aren't particularly overcome with desire for sexual activity, you should make a special effort to indulge regularly whenever possible. Many "sexually inactive" people who make an effort to resume sexual activities are surprised to find that they can once again enjoy the pleasures of sex. Take the case of Mary Ann C., for example. She was not very active sexually after her menopause. When her husband became impotent because of a prostate disorder, she became *totally* inactive. She was 60 years of age when her husband died. "My life is nearly over," she said, "and I have nothing to live for. My health is too bad to allow me to go back to work."

Mary Ann eventually met a retired business executive and fell in love. Almost immediately, her health improved and her sexual desire returned. When her romance led to marriage, she was astonished to find that she could once again reach a climax during intercourse. "I thought I was sexually dead," she whispered to friends. "But now it seems that I have been sexually revived. And I feel better than I have felt in years."

It's becoming more and more apparent to physicians that romance improves the health of older persons. A happy sex life at any age can do wonders in maintaining emotional balance. Many "nervous disorders" can be traced to loneliness or sexual frustration.

Single persons who do not have sexual partners should feel free to indulge in masturbation or self relief when they are so inclined. No harm will result from self relief, and no effort should be made to refrain when the desire is present. Unrelieved sexual tension at any age can be harmful.

Pornography Isn't All Bad!

If you feel that the use of "pornography" helps you in the performance or enjoyment of sex, then by all means use it. There isn't anything wrong with looking at pictures or movies portraying normal sexual activities. I have heard of many cases in which the use of instructional "pornography" revived marriages and brought new pleasure to an otherwise stale or inhibited partnership.

MENOPAUSE:
THE BEGINNING OF A NEW LIFE

Contrary to popular belief, menopause in the female does not mean that her sexual desires will automatically diminish. In fact, more often than not, menopause contributed to an *increase* in sexual desire by removing the fear of pregnancy. If a woman is convinced, however, that menopause represents the end of her sex life, she may develop a mental barrier that will indeed bring her sex life to an end. And if she allows her physical condition to "go to pot," she may no longer interest her husband. This creates a vicious cycle in which "frigidity" and "impotence" lead to physical deterioration and a sexually dead marriage.

Almost without exception, couples who remain sexually

active late in life do so because *both* partners continue to express an interest in each other. When one partner is uncooperative, unwilling, or always complaining, there may not be sufficient stimulation to bring about a sexual union. When this happens, a marriage dies physically, with both partners placing the blame on "old age." You don't have to let that happen to you.

STAY PHYSICALLY ATTRACTIVE

Although most people like to believe that love is a spiritual thing that does not depend upon physical beauty, it's undeniably true that sexual love is considerably enhanced by physical beauty. Try to keep your body lean, clean, and attractively clothed. Do the best you can to *look* sexy. It'll pay big dividends in arousing the interest of the opposite sex.

Many men and women who assume that their mates are sexually dead are shocked to learn that a spouse is "having an affair." In many of these cases, the adulterer is literally driven into the arms of someone who stimulates or encourages them. It's important to remember that some older men cannot *perform* sexually without adequate psychological and physical stimulation. A woman can always *perform,* but she cannot *respond* without being prepared mentally. So it's important for both man and wife to do all they can physically and mentally to stimulate each other sexually.

GOOD HEALTH IS ESSENTIAL
FOR SEXUAL HAPPINESS

No matter how ambitious you might be about remaining sexually active late in life, you won't be able to perform if you aren't in fairly good health. Chronic fatigue, for example, which is often the result of nutritional deficiency, is a common cause of sexual inactivity. So be sure to eat properly. A balanced diet of fresh, natural foods that includes the use of such basic food supplements as brewer's yeast, desiccated liver, and wheat germ will contribute to sexual vigor and help prevent fatigue and illness.

How to Use Vitamin E
to Increase Sexual Vigor

If you're a little low on vigor and you feel that you need a boost, you may be able to get the help you need from Vitamin E. Some researchers now maintain that Vitamin E contributes greatly to sexual endurance. It's well known that it increases *physical* endurance by reducing the body's need for oxygen. Vitamin E also improves circulation and increases the oxygen-carrying capacity of the blood. There is even some evidence to indicate that it will delay the aging process by preventing oxidation of tissue cells and essential fatty acids.

Vitamin E certainly won't do any harm — and if it doesn't help your sex life it might help your heart and your blood vessels. You'll learn more about Vitamin E and the heart under Life Extender #4.

The minimum daily requirement for Vitamin E is usually given as 30 international units. Nutritionists tell us that the average American diet, which is made up largely of refined foods, supplies only about 12 units. So in order to get the amount of Vitamin E you need for exceptional vigor and endurance, you may have to make use of special supplements.

Wheat germ and wheat germ oil are the best natural sources of Vitamin E. A teaspoonful of wheat germ oil, however, contains only about 10 units of Vitamin E — and you may need a *few hundred* units daily for good results. I usually recommend about 400 units for females and 600 units for males. It's probably best to divide this amount into three doses, one about 15 minutes *before* each meal.

If you have high blood pressure, begin with 100 units daily and increase the amount about 100 units a week until a maximum dose of about 400 units is reached. Have your blood pressure checked regularly; if it shows a progressive rise, it might be necessary to reduce your intake of Vitamin E to about 100 units daily. If you have a rheumatic heart, you may have to be cautious about taking large doses of Vitamin E. Check with your doctor.

Natural Vitamin E is about five times more potent than synthetic Vitamin E. So be sure to pick a natural brand, even if it costs a little more.

How to Increase Physical
Endurance with Wheat Germ Oil

Even if you take a Vitamin E supplement, you should include a little wheat germ oil in your diet. The studies of Dr. Thomas Cureton of the University of Illinois showed that a group of men who took one teaspoonful of wheat germ oil daily while training on a treadmill had *51 percent more endurance* than a group that trained without taking the oil. This was believed to be due more to other substances in the oil than to Vitamin E.

In a similar test involving two groups of middle-aged men, the group that took wheat germ oil was proved by scientific tests to have greater endurance and stamina. They also had less heart stress and quicker body reaction.

To be sure of getting all the benefits of wheat germ oil, use a tablespoonful daily on a fresh green salad — or simply mix the oil into appropriate foods.

The stamina and increased endurance that result from Vitamin E and wheat germ oil are bound to contribute to improved sexual performance. They will certainly improve your health.

INSTANT ENERGY FOR SEX

You've heard it said many times that a cold shower cools sexual ardor. If you're short on energy for lovemaking, however, proper use of cold water can charge you with the energy you need for sexual activities. Too much cold will leave you fatigued, but short applications of cold should prove to be stimulating.

Few people can step into a cold shower. It's usually best to begin with a *warm* shower and then gradually turn it down to a comfortably cold temperature. If such a shower does not leave you feeling warm and energetic, it means that either the water was too cold or you stayed in the shower too long. You should never use water so cold that you feel chilled after leaving the shower.

Remember that a cold shower will wake you up and stimulate your nervous system, while a warm shower will relax you or put you to sleep.

How to Use a Wet-Sheet
Rub for Mutual Stimulation

The wet-sheet rub is probably the most effective tonic a couple can use for mutual stimulation. All you have to do is wrap your partner in a cool, wet sheet and rub vigorously — and then take the treatment yourself.

Sheet rub technique. Strip down to your birthday suit. Wring a sheet out in cold water (60 to 70 degrees Fahrenheit) and stand erect so that the sheet can be wrapped around you in the following manner:

Hold up both of your arms. Place the upper corner of one side of the sheet under your left arm and then lower that arm to hold the sheet in place. Have your partner wrap the sheet around your chest and back and then lower your right arm. The sheet is then wrapped *over* your arms, chest, and shoulders and around your neck so that it can be tucked under the edge of the sheet behind your neck.

Instruct your partner to rub and slap the sheet vigorously over your entire body until the sheet becomes warm. The trick is to rub the sheet without making it slide over the skin.

Dry your body by replacing the wet sheet with a warm, dry sheet for a dry-sheet rub. Use the same wrapping and rubbing technique used in the wet-sheet rub. Finish by rubbing your body vigorously with a coarse towel.

I recently recommended the wet-sheet rub for a couple who admitted that they both were usually "too tired" to make love. Part of the husband's trouble was a bad habit of overeating at night. He was so stuffed at bedtime that he could do little but flop down and go to sleep. The wife was so accustomed to being neglected that she made no effort to prepare herself for possible lovemaking. Instead, she usually retired in a faded, baggy nightgown that made her shapeless and unappealing. I advised the husband to eat less at night and to try the wet-sheet rub with his wife after their evening bath. The very next day, the husband reported that the experiment was a great success. "We both rediscovered our bodies," he said with obvious delight. "And the tonic effect of the wet sheet really got us going!"

**How to Use
a Sitting Water Tonic**

A cold *sitz bath* may help stimulate waning sexual powers. Put about four inches of cold water in a large pan and then sit in the water for a few minutes. You can measure four inches of water by touching the bottom of the pan with the tip of your index finger. If the water reaches your knuckles, you have four inches of water. Sitting in cold water will result in a circulatory reaction that will gorge the pelvic area with blood as well as stimulate nerves.

For a colder, more stimulating sitz bath, put a few ice cubes in a bath tub containing four inches of water and then sit in it with your knees bent so that only your buttocks and your feet are submerged. Sit in the water for at least 15 minutes.

While you're sitting in cold water, contraction of the blood vessels in the pelvic area will reduce the flow of blood to the sexual organs. This won't result in any immediate sexual stimulation. The toning effect that cold water has on the blood vessels, however, will contribute to improved sexual performance later.

Special Foods for Male Vigor

Since a man's semen is composed largely of lecithin, the same substance that dissolves hard fat in the arteries, every male over the age of forty should probably add lecithin to his diet. It can be sprinkled over foods as granules or taken in tablet form.

Seminal fluid also contains zinc and magnesium, which can be supplied by wheat germ, beef liver, oysters, nuts, seeds, and whole grains. Vitamin F and raw pumpkin seeds have been found to be beneficial in the treatment of prostate troubles.

The amino acids glycine, alanine, and glutamic acid, found in protein-rich foods, are essential for a healthy prostate gland.

Always make sure that your diet contains adequate protein. Baked chicken, broiled fish, and cottage cheese are good sources of low-fat protein for rebuilding aging and deteriorating tissues.

HOW TO CHARGE MALE
BATTERIES WITH A HEALTHY PROSTATE

The prostate gland has a lot to do with male sexual potency. When a man begins to lose his sexual powers, he begins to feel old. His youth battery is clearly running down, and chances are his prostate gland is weak and unhealthy.

A zinc deficiency is sometimes a factor in the development of prostate trouble. It's well known that the prostate gland normally contains more zinc than any other part of the body. The fluid secreted by the prostate also contains a large amount of zinc. When there is a zinc deficiency, the prostate gland enlarges and does not produce adequate amounts of prostatic fluid. This results in a decrease in sexual desire, along with a drop in drive, vitality, and general health. It has been estimated that about seven percent of healthy males have a prostatic zinc deficiency, with about 30 percent showing a borderline deficiency. Enlargement of the prostate gland is common after middle age, with at least one out of every three men suffering from prostate trouble. So it might be a good idea to make sure that your diet contains adequate zinc.

Oysters, meats, nuts, whole wheat, lima beans, dried green peas, rye seeds, nonfat dry milk, eggs, chicken, and brewer's yeast are good sources of zinc. Fresh oysters are the richest source of zinc, since they contain 1,487 parts per million of zinc compared with 56.6 parts per million in round steak, the next richest source.

When there is a zinc deficiency because of poor intestinal absorption, it may be necessary to take a zinc supplement, such as zinc gluconate. Good results have been achieved with 50 to 220 milligrams of zinc daily.

A Test for Prostate Infection

When the prostate gland is infected, there may be backache, fever, and other symptoms, such as pain on ejaculation.

Collect a urine specimen (in a clean glass) at the end of urination and hold it up to the light and look for cloudiness. If the prostate is infected, the urine will be very cloudy. See your doctor for diagnosis and treatment.

Relief for Prostate Trouble

Prostate trouble is a common complaint among men who are over forty years of age. For some reason, the prostate gland of an aging man almost always enlarges enough to cause trouble. And when it does, difficulty emptying the bladder is one of the first symptoms. "I have to get up several times every night to go to the bathroom just to dribble a small amount of urine," complained Arnold T., a victim of prostate trouble.

I explained to Arnold that a hot sitz bath provides the most effective treatment for simple swelling of the prostate gland. "All you have to do," I explained, "is run about four inches of comfortably hot water into a tub or pan and then sit in the water for about ten minutes each night. Be sure to empty your bladder before going to bed."

A few weeks later, Arnold reported that he could empty his bladder much better. "I only have to get up once or twice a night now," he said, "instead of seven or eight times."

Most natural remedies are as effective as they are simple. So don't fail to try a remedy just because it isn't complicated or difficult to use. Simple moist heat, for example, is one of the most effective and readily available remedies I know of for relieving the symptoms of a great variety of ailments — including prostate trouble.

HOW TO RELIEVE
MENOPAUSAL VAGINITIS

After menopause, a woman's ovaries cease producing estrogen. This sometimes allows the development of vaginitis, a dry vaginal inflammation that makes intercourse painful. A gynecologist can prescribe vaginal creams containing estrogen, or natural estrogen in tablet form for oral use. Oral estrogen is just as effective as injected estrogen. So ask your doctor for estrogen *tablets* in order to avoid frequent trips to a doctor's office. If you have even had a tumor or a malignancy, you should not take estrogen in any form.

Vitamin E has been found to be useful in overcoming chronic vaginitis. Try taking a hundred units daily and then slowly increase the dosage to about 400 units.

How to Take
a Vinegar Douche

The vagina is normally acid, but when inflammation or infection is present it is often found to be alkaline. A series of vinegar douches will help restore vaginal acidity. Add three tablespoons of white vinegar or one teaspoonful of lactic acid to two quarts of water and douche daily until the infection is gone. Each time you douche, be sure to hold the water in with hand pressure until the vagina is full and then suddenly release the water. Repeat this procedure until you have used two quarts of water.

If vaginal infection persists, a gynecologist can prescribe suppositories that can be converted to lactic acid by bacterial action in the vagina.

A NEED TO BE LOVED

Everyone wants to be touched and loved. A hug, a pat, or just a warm closeness, with or without sex, helps to fulfill a human need for affection. So even if you are not sexually active, you should continue to exchange affection with your mate. Nothing causes more unhappiness than isolation that cuts off a close, warm relationship with other human beings. So don't be afraid to show your feelings for someone you love. Remember that you must give love in order to receive love. In many cases, a simple exchange of affection can revive a marriage and give new meaning to life.

Jack and Lucille had a cold marriage and a business-like relationship. Neither felt that it was necessary to "prove" their love for each other. As a result, Lucille never received much attention, so she refrained from displays of affection for Jack. Their marriage was physically dead. When Lucille began to suffer from a variety of vague nervous complaints, I suggested to Jack that perhaps she was suffering from doubts about her feminine appeal. Actually, she was suffering from lack of love. When Jack was persuaded to display a little affection for Lucille, she responded immediately. In a few weeks, she was transformed from a "sick old woman" to a radiant, relaxed, and confident wife.

"I thought my husband didn't love me," Lucille confessed, "and I felt so useless and unwanted." Jack admitted that for the first time in years they had an active sex life.

There are many people who have problems which could be solved with a little love and affection.

Summary

1. All available evidence indicates that most people can enjoy sexual activities well into their eighties and beyond.
2. It's now well known that the more active a person is sexually the longer he will keep his sexual powers.
3. Mental attitude, physical appearance, and a willing partner have a lot to do with sexual success in marriage.
4. Menopause should contribute to sexual enjoyment by removing the fear of pregnancy.
5. Vitamin E and wheat germ oil can increase sexual power by increasing physical endurance.
6. The wet-sheet rub described in this chapter is an effective way to generate energy for sexual activity.
7. Pumpkin seeds, wheat germ, beef liver, oysters, nuts, seeds, and whole grains supply food elements that are essential for a healthy prostate gland.
8. Inflammation of the prostate gland can be relieved by sitting in four inches of comfortably hot water.

9. Natural estrogen tablets, taken orally, or vaginal creams containing estrogen, may be helpful in overcoming the dry inflammation of menopausal vaginitis.

10. Remember that you must give love to receive love. Don't be reluctant to show affection for someone you love.

LIFE EXTENDER #4

How to Revitalize
Body Functions and
Re-Energize Vital Organs

In the opening pages of this book, you learned that practically everyone dies of disease rather than old age. If you practice good nutrition and take good care of yourself, your chances of living a long, healthy life will be good. As you grow older, however, your body functions tend to slow down, and your organs do not generate the power they once did. Although this deterioration is a gradual process that begins early in life, it always seems to strike suddenly in middle age. The age of 40, for example, is commonly thought of as a starting point for the aches and pains of aging.

There's much that you can do at home to relieve the various ailments that are associated with the aging process. You'll learn more about home remedies in other portions of this book. With Life Extender #4, you'll learn how to stimulate your body and strengthen your organs so that you can combat the aging process and feel better. Some of the measures are so simple and so effective that you'll want to use them every day of your life. Did you know, for example, that rocking in a rocking chair aids the function of the heart? Or that deep breathing aids the circulation of blood? You can actually *measure* the strength of your heart with a simple record of your pulse rate. Proper selection of foods will combat heart disease and hardening of the arteries. You can use sleep, water, massage, sunshine, posture, and food supplements to rejuvenate your body and prolong your life. These and other secrets of good health and longevity are yours for the reading.

HOW TO BREATHE NEW
LIFE INTO YOUR BODY

Shortness of breath is one of the first symptoms we notice when we begin to feel "old." There are several reasons for this. One is that the body is in such poor physical condition that even a small amount of physical activity demands a large amount of oxygen. Another is that the heart and lungs perform so inefficiently that they must labor to meet the demands of the slightest exertion. Chronic ailments such as anemia, emphysema, and hardened arteries can interfere with the function of the heart and the lungs.

You can actually exercise your lungs with simple breathing exercises. And in doing so, you can aid your heart in the circulation of blood.

How to Breathe Deeply Safely

Since your lungs are composed of lobes containing millions of tiny air sacs, you must make a special effort to make sure that *all* of the sacs are occasionally expanded in order to remove stale air and to open the channels between your lungs and your blood vessels. To do this, you'll have to take a couple of special exercises. This means combining forced deep breathing with such simple exercises as walking or bicycling.

In forced deep breathing, there are a few precautions that must be observed. One is that you should always stop your breathing exercises when you begin to feel dizzy. Prolonged, forced deep breathing when there is not a demand for oxygen can constrict the blood vessels around your brain by siphoning too much carbon dioxide out of your blood.

The best time to take breathing exercises is after walking or exerting yourself, when you are a little breathless. Otherwise, you should limit your deep breathing to a couple of deep breaths at a time. I'd recommend that you take your breathing exercises in a sitting position. Then, if you should become dizzy from hyperventilation, you won't fall and hurt yourself. Just sit erect in a chair, place your hands on your knees, and then press lightly against your knees while you inhale deeply. Lift your chest as high as you can with each breath. This simple posture will anchor your shoulder blades so that certain chest muscles can be used to lift your rib cage.

**Abdominal Breathing
Is Also Important**

Occasionally inhale deeply into your abdomen to make a "pot belly." Then exhale and contract your abdominal muscles. Remember that it's just as important to strengthen your abdominal muscles as it is to strengthen your chest muscles when you do breathing exercises.

When your breathing is relaxed, your diaphragm works automatically in a form of abdominal breathing. When you are breathless, your diaphragm and your chest and abdominal muscles work together to fully expand the upper and lower lobes of your lungs. If all these muscles have been strengthened by breathing exercises, the lungs can function much better in overcoming the effects of emphysema and other aging respiratory ailments.

**Breathing Aids the
Circulation of Blood**

Rhythmical breathing aids the circulation of blood by creating a suction effect that pulls blood up through the big veins below the heart. When you breathe deeply during and after exercise, you can take advantage of your breathlessness to force maximum expansion of your lungs. And in doing so, you increase the flow of blood as well as the supply of oxygen to muscles and organs. There's one special precaution, however, that you must *always* observe when you combine exercise and deep breathing: you should *never* take a deep breath and hold

it during an exertion. Holding your breath while you are straining creates positive pressure in your chest and abdomen and
may interfere with the circulation of blood enough to cause a
blackout. Always breathe rhythmically when you exercise,
and always exhale during a heavy exertion.

HOW TO EAT TO
ENRICH YOUR BLOOD

No matter how efficiently you breathe, you must have good,
rich blood to absorb oxygen in your lungs and to "service" the
tissues of your body. This means that you must have an adequate number of iron-rich blood cells. You can supply your
blood cells with iron by eating generous amounts of dark-green
leafy vegetables, dried fruit, and lean meats. Wheat germ,
brewer's yeast, and blackstrap molasses are highly concentrated sources of iron.

You also need plenty of protein and Vitamin B_{12} to build
blood cells. Liver is the best source of Vitamin B_{12}, and, like
any meat, is a good source of protein. Since liver is rich in
cholesterol, however, you probably shouldn't eat it more often
than once a week if your blood cholesterol is high. All foods of
animal origin contain some Vitamin B_{12}. If you eat eggs,
cheese, fish, or meat each day, or if you drink milk, you'll
probably get adequate amounts of B_{12} for blood-building
purposes.

Note: Since Vitamin B_{12} is found almost exclusively in foods
of animal origin, it's not a good idea to go on a strict vege-
tarian diet. Your intestinal tract manufactures some B_{12}, but
not enough to do without animal products. If you don't eat
meat or fish, you should at least eat eggs and cheese or drink
milk — or take a Vitamin B_{12} supplement.

Although vegetables do not contain Vitamin B_{12}, they do
contain folic acid, a B vitamin which helps manufacture blood
cells. But when there is a Vitamin B_{12} deficiency, the folic acid
will sometimes mask the deficiency until permanent damage
occurs in the nervous system. So in order to make sure that
your blood cells and your nervous system have an adequate

amount of Vitamin B_{12}, you should eat some animal products each day, no matter how good you feel on a diet of fruits and vegetables.

Stomach Acid Helps
Prevent Anemia

It's well known that stomach acid is needed for the absorption of iron and Vitamin B_{12}. It's also well known that persons over 40 tend to be *deficient* in stomach acid. The B vitamins in the foods you eat help your body manufacture hydrochloric acid for your stomach, but it might be a good idea to try taking a hydrochloric acid supplement if you are anemic and you are having digestive troubles. You can purchase such a supplement in drug stores and in health food stores.

Jason E. had always been a little anemic, and he suffered constantly from sour stomach, belching, and other symptoms of "indigestion." He was constantly taking alkalizers, but his indigestion grew worse. And in spite of eating iron-rich foods, he remained anemic. Since Jason was in his late sixties, I suggested that perhaps he should discontinue the alkalizers and try taking hydrochloric acid tablets. "No harm would result," I assured him. "If your indigestion improves, you can continue taking the tablets. If your indigestion grows worse, you can quit taking the tablets."

Jason took the tablets as I suggested. He experienced immediate relief from his indigestion. His blood picture also improved, and it appeared that his hemoglobin and cell count would eventually return to normal. No amount of food would have accomplished the task without an acid supplement to aid in the absorption of iron and Vitamin B_{12}.

Note: When anemia occurs in spite of a good, balanced diet and adequate stomach acid, the stomach may be deficient in an "intrinsic substance" needed for the absorption of Vitamin B_{12}. When this is the case, a physician may have to inject the vitamin into the body. Special blood studies will reveal the need for such injections.

HOW TO KEEP YOUR ARTERIES
YOUTHFUL FOR A LONGER LIFE

For good circulation, you must have good arteries. Unfortunately, poor circulation is one of the hazards of aging. Hardened arteries, or arteries clogged with hard fat and cholesterol, play havoc with the flow of blood to important organs. Each year, more than 700,000 Americans die from heart attacks, largely because of diseased arteries. Many factors play a part in the development of clogged arteries. Dietary factors are probably most important. Fortunately, there are some simple dietary programs that anyone can follow to relieve or reverse the effects of hard, clogged arteries.

Note: Women are less subject to hardening of the arteries until after menopause, when they lose protection afforded by certain female hormones.

How to Control the Fat in
Your Diet for Healthy Arteries

Most nutrition authorities now believe that an excessive amount of animal fat in the diet contributes to the development of hardened arteries. And at least one cancer researcher has linked colon cancer to excessive use of fatty foods. So it's generally recommended that everyone go easy on meat fat, butter, grease, whole milk products, and other foods that are rich in saturated fat and cholesterol, such as organ meats and shell fish.

Egg yolk is rich in cholesterol. But if eggs are soft boiled so that the yolk remains a little runny, the lecithin and essential fatty acids in the yolk will counteract the cholesterol. Many physicians recommend that you not eat more than two or three egg yolks a week. If you eat a balanced diet of natural foods, however, rich in B vitamins, I personally do not feel that an egg a day would be harmful. Quite the contrary, if you reduce your intake of other foods that are rich in saturated fat and cholesterol, it's not likely that you'll get too much cholesterol from properly prepared eggs. The yolk of an egg is rich in iron, Vitamin A, essential fatty acids, and other nutrients needed for good health and a long life. The white of an egg is almost pure protein.

The fat in whole milk is a saturated variety that contributes to the formation of hard fat in the arteries. If you drink large quantities of milk, you should drink skim milk most of the time. Cottage cheese made from skim milk supplies most of the nutrients of milk, minus the fat.

A small amount of butter may be beneficial to health, since it supplies essential nutrients and aids in the absorption of Vitamins A and D. A little butter on toast is all right occasionally, but you should not eat butter at every meal or put it in other foods.

There must always be a certain amount of fat in your diet for good health. So it isn't necessary to avoid fat completely. The trick is to *reduce* the amount of animal fat in your diet and then balance it with an equal amount of vegetable fat. This will keep the saturated fat and cholesterol in your arteries from becoming hard.

Remember, however, that all fats and oils contain a lot of calories. So while it's important to use a little vegetable oil in cooking and on your salads, you shouldn't use any more than necessary to counteract the small amount of animal fat in your diet. A couple tablespoons of cold-pressed safflower oil, wheat germ oil, or corn oil daily on a green salad will be enough if you eat properly. You shouldn't eat fried foods very often, but when you do you should use vegetable oil instead of butter, lard, or bacon grease for frying. Vegetable oil should also be used in baking whenever possible.

Remember this important rule: Cut down the total amount of fat in your diet so that you get only about 25 percent of your calories from fat, with one-half to two-thirds of them coming from vegetable sources.

How to Use B Vitamins to Combat Hardening of the Arteries

Plenty of B vitamins will help your body manufacture lecithin and other substances you need to keep the cholesterol in your blood from clogging your arteries. Choline, inositol, niacin, and pyridoxin, for example, have been found to be helpful in combating hardening of the arteries. Brewer's yeast, wheat germ, and desiccated liver are good sources of all the B vitamins.

Contrary to popular belief, cholesterol is essential for good health. Your body actually manufactures it. Too much cholesterol in the diet, however, when combined with a deficiency in certain essential nutrients, results in hardened or clogged arteries. Just try to follow a sensible, balanced diet. Remember that excesses of any kind create imbalances that may be harmful to your health.

Is Your Cholesterol Normal?

Most doctors consider a blood cholesterol level of 150 to 250 milligrams per 100 cubic centimeters of blood to be normal. Remember, however, that it's also considered "normal" to die at about 70 years of age. With most people dying from heart disease or suffering from clogged arteries, you cannot be guided by the standards of the average person. If your own blood cholesterol is above 180 milligrams percent, it may be too high to assure youthful arteries for a long life. So don't be encouraged to continue with bad eating habits just because your blood cholesterol is "not above normal." It's also important to make sure that the hard fat (lipoprotein and triglyceride) level of your blood is not too high. All this can be checked with a single blood sample from your arm.

Sugar and White Flour
Can Damage Your Arteries

There is now some evidence to indicate that excessive use of sugar and white flour products may be a leading cause of clogged arteries. They certainly contribute to a build-up of hard fat and cholesterol in the blood. Cut down on them as much as possible. Sugar may actually *steal* the B vitamins your body needs to combat atherosclerosis. It may also contribute to the development of diabetes, which can seriously complicate arterial disease and circulatory problems.

How Vitamin E
Helps Your Blood Vessels

Vitamin E is often used in the treatment of diseases of the heart and blood vessels. It's believed that this important vitamin dilates blood vessels and helps prevent the formation of clots inside the arteries. Vitamin E also reduces the body's need for oxygen, making it possible for the body to function normally in spite of hardened arteries. Leg cramps caused by poor circulation, for example, can often be relieved with Vitamin E. The older you become the more important it is to take a Vitamin E supplement. But don't wait too long. Remember that Vitamin E delays the aging process and combats atherosclerosis by preventing oxidation of the essential fatty acids.

Most Vitamin E comes in the form of oil that has been distilled from vegetable oil or wheat germ oil. If you can't tolerate oil, you can purchase special Vitamin E wafers in health food stores.

WHAT TO DO ABOUT LEG ACHE
CAUSED BY HARDENED ARTERIES

One of the first symptoms of arteriosclerosis or hardened arteries is leg ache or "intermittent claudication." This means that the circulation of blood to the leg muscles is so poor that walking causes an oxygen deficiency that results in cramping or aching. The aching is relieved by rest but returns again when walking is resumed. Although walking triggers the aching, it's important to take regular walking exercises. Just walk until the aching begins, rest, and then resume walking. Combining walking exercise with Vitamin E and other dietary measures will increase the distance you can walk without pain. Contraction of leg muscles during walking will pump blood through the legs, while the Vitamin E helps open the arteries.

Frank K. was sixty-one when he started having trouble with his legs. "When I sold my package store and retired," he related, "I started doing a little hunting and discovered that I couldn't walk very far without having bad leg cramps." I advised Frank to start taking 600 units of Vitamin E daily and to walk every day until his legs started to ache. Several weeks later, he reported that he could walk about a mile without any trouble. Chances are Frank will eventually be able to walk as far as he wants to on a long hunting trip if he continues with his Vitamin E and his walking exercise.

**How to Aid Venous and
Arterial Blood Flow in Your Legs**

When *hardened arteries* cause leg pain while walking, the
pain must be relieved by *rest*. But when the pain occurs while
resting in bed, it can usually be relieved by walking. So if you
have hardened arteries and poor circulation and you develop
leg ache or cramping at night, just get out of bed and walk
around a little. Or simply sit on the side of the bed with your
legs hanging down and flex your ankles back and forth. In
either case, muscle contraction and the pull of gravity will
increase the flow of blood through hardened arteries. Persons
who suffer from nightly leg ache caused by hardened arteries
are often advised to place a brick under each head post of their
bed in order to aid arterial blood flow while they sleep.

Persons who suffer from leg ache caused by *varicose veins*
can often relieve their symptoms by *elevating* their legs — or
by wrapping their legs with an elastic bandage to prevent venous
congestion. (See Life Extender #10 for additional information
on how to care for varicose veins.)

There's a simple exercise that you can do to aid the flow of
blood in both the veins and the arteries of your legs. Lie on
your back on a bed that has a brick under the head posts. Alternately raise and lower one leg at a time. When the leg goes
up, the venous blood will be drained. When the leg is lowered,
the flow of blood in the arteries will increase. This exercise simply uses the pull of gravity to fill and empty the veins and arteries.

**How to Revive
Your Body with Water**

Applying water to your body is a good way to stimulate the
circulation of blood. When you take a hot bath, for example,
the blood vessels in your skin dilate and draw blood to the
surface to keep your body temperature from rising. Cold water
constricts the blood vessels of the skin and drives blood inward in order to conserve body temperature. You can actually
exercise your blood vessels and your circulation by taking a
hot bath followed by a warm shower that's gradually turned
down to a comfortably cold temperature.

A brisk towel rub or a rubdown following a cold shower should leave your skin glowing with warmth.

Note: Warm water relaxes the body, while cold water stimulates the body. When you want to relax and retire for the evening, simply take a warm tub bath and go to bed. When you need a little wide-awake energy, however, get under a cool shower and then gradually turn it down until it's as cold as you can stand it. Rub your body vigorously with both hands while the temperature of the water is being lowered. Remember that only a brief exposure to cold water is needed for a tonic effect. Too long an exposure may result in fatigue.

As you grow older, your body will not react as well to cold water as it did when you were younger. So be sure not to use water so cold that it produces a chill.

**Hydrovascular Exercise
for Fun and Fitness**

Exercising in water offers a potent form of circulatory stimulation. The buoyancy of the water will aid the flow of venous blood through the legs, while contraction of the muscles will pump blood through veins and arteries. The antigravity effects of water submersion will also relieve the pull on muscles, joints, and organs. Just stand in neck deep water and move your arms and legs through the water as rapidly as possible. The resistance of the water will provide plenty of exercise for your muscles, and the combined effects of muscle contraction and water pressure will greatly aid circulation.

HOW TO TEST YOUR HEART
BY TESTING YOUR PULSE

Heart muscle is similar to skeletal muscle. Both become weak when they are not exercised. You can measure the strength of your heart by taking your pulse. If your resting pulse rate is high, or considerably above 72, this may mean that the heart muscle is not pumping an adequate amount of blood with each contraction and must beat rapidly to pump enough blood to meet the demands of your body.

At 70 beats per minute and a half-second pause between beats, the work your heart does is balanced by an equal amount of rest. When your pulse rate goes up, however, your heart works more than it rests. A low pulse rate, on the other hand, gives your heart more time to rest and repair itself.

Some type of regular exercise, such as walking, swimming, or riding a bicycle, will strengthen your heart muscle, lower your pulse rate, and improve circulation. Whatever type of exercise you do, always exercise until you are short of breath or until your pulse rate has increased considerably. It takes several minutes of endurance-type exercise to have a training effect on the heart. Don't push yourself, however. Keep your effort well within a range of comfort. Always stop when you begin to feel uncomfortable. If you exercise regularly, at least every other day, you'll gradually increase your capacity for exercise, and your heart and lungs will become progressively stronger.

I discovered during a routine physical examination that George J. had a resting pulse rate of about 120. After only a few minutes of simple test exercises, he was puffing from exhaustion. And after five minutes of rest, his heart rate was still considerably higher than his resting rate. Since George was flabby and overweight, it was apparent that he was simply in poor physical condition. Special tests by his family physician had already ruled out any heart or thyroid abnormality. So I started him on a physical training program that began with simple walking. By the end of the sixth week, George was alternately walking and jogging about a mile every other day. When I saw him six months later, his resting pulse rate was only 70, and he had lost nearly all of his excess body weight. "I feel much better now," he confessed. "Life is a lot easier for me, and I'm getting much more work done."

A strong heart and a lower pulse rate will prolong your life as well as take the strain out of living. No matter what your goals in life might be, you'll have a better chance of reaching them with a low pulse rate.

Start keeping a record of your pulse rate and see if it doesn't get lower after you have been exercising for several weeks. When your resting pulse rate drops to 65 or lower, you'll know that your heart muscle is in good condition.

You can double check your heart by taking your pulse rate while lying down and while standing erect. If there is a difference of more than 15 to 20 beats per minute, it may mean that your heart is still not as strong as it should be.

Note: Coffee, tea, cocoa, and cola drinks contain caffeine that will increase your pulse rate. You shouldn't drink these beverages at all if your pulse rate is consistently above 80 or if your heart is always "skipping beats."

How to Take Your Pulse

It's a simple matter to take your pulse. All you have to do is place the fingertips of your right hand over the thumbside of the inside portion of your left wrist. Count your pulse rate for 15 seconds and multiply by four to get the rate per minute. Remember that your heart beats faster after eating. So be sure to take your pulse *before* you eat.

Walk to Save Your Legs

There's an old saying that if you don't use your legs you'll lose them. Without muscle contraction to pump blood through the legs, the arteries and veins of the legs tend to become clogged and inflamed. This can lead to the formation of blood clots that can cause disability or even loss of a leg. So even if you're not concerned about your heart, you should exercise your legs regularly by walking or riding a bicycle.

HOW TO HELP YOUR HEART WITH A ROCKING CHAIR

When you aren't able to walk for some reason, or if you are forced to sit for long periods of time, you should rock in a rocking chair. The rhythmical to and fro motion of rocking forces the muscles of the body to contract and relax so that they act as subsidiary pumps in the movement of blood. In this way, a rocking chair actually helps the heart. So don't just sit. Rock!

HOW TO IMPROVE CIRCULATION
WITH A SLANT BOARD

As we grow older, the blood supply to the brain tends to diminish because of hardened arteries, making it increasingly more difficult to concentrate or remember.

A slant board can be used to improve the flow of blood to the brain. All you have to do is get a board that's wide enough and long enough to support your body from head to foot. Just prop one end of the board up on a chair and lie down on the board with your feet anchored at the high end of the board. This upside down position will reverse the effects of gravity, draining venous blood out of the legs and increasing the flow of arterial blood to the brain. In addition to clearing the brain and relieving leg ache caused by varicose veins, lying on a slant board will relieve pressure on spinal joints and discs. It will also shift pressures on sagging abdominal organs.

Note: If you have high blood pressure, or if you have head-aches often, you may have to limit elevation of the board to 12 inches or less. Whatever height you use, don't continue to lie on the board after you begin to feel uncomfortable. Remember that legs crippled by hardened arteries are best relieved by *lowering* the legs. Also, the heart must work harder to pump blood through the legs in an upside down position. So if you suffer from clogged or diseased leg arteries, or if you have a weak heart, don't lie on a slant board very long, and don't use a steep incline.

HOW TO LENGTHEN YOUR
LIFE WITH SLEEP

The recovery and healing powers of your body depend great-ly upon getting adequate sleep. Chronic loss of sleep can lead to fatigue, disease, infection, and premature aging. Too much sleep, however, may be equally harmful. There is some evi-dence, for example, to indicate that *persons who average seven to eight hours of sleep each night have the longest life expec-*

tancy, while persons who sleep *long* hours are more susceptible to certain types of disease. A six-year study by one doctor, for example, revealed that men in their fifties who sleep nine hours or more each night have twice as many strokes, heart attacks, and aneurysms as those who sleep seven hours or less. And the longer they sleep the greater the risk. One reason for this is that prolonged immobility slows the circulation and allows the development of circulatory problems. So while you need *adequate* sleep to replenish energy stores and to give your body a chance to repair and replace wornout tissue cells, an excessive amount of sleep may result in physical and mental sluggishness that will weaken the body's defense against disease.

As you grow older, you may need more sleep than you did when you were younger. Persons over 60 years of age, for example, may need as much as ten hours of sleep each night, with a one-hour nap in the afternoon. Rather than stay in bed for ten hours, however, it might be best to sleep several hours at night and then catch a few naps during the day. This will prevent excessive circulatory stagnation.

Be guided by the way you feel in deciding how much sleep is best for you. Get the sleep you need but don't lie in bed and *try* to sleep just to pass the time. If you go to bed at the same time each night, chances are you'll wake up at the same time each morning. Once you know how much sleep you need, you can get in and out of bed with consistent regularity.

Hints for Sounder Sleep

Regular sleeping hours. Go to bed at the same time each night. Once you become accustomed to regular sleeping hours, you won't have any trouble falling asleep each night. Best of all, you'll wake up at the same time each morning, refreshed and ready to begin the day.

The first four hours of sleep are the deepest and the most important. If noise, visitors, or some other unexpected disturbance keeps you awake the first half of the night, you may not be able to catch up on your sleep by sleeping a few extra hours in the morning. In this case, a short nap during the day may be beneficial. Remember, however, that if you sleep too much during the day you should not expect to be able to sleep at night.

Night sleeping is best. Daytime sleeping may not be as deep and restful as nighttime sleeping, especially if you are accustomed to sleeping at night. The noise of people and machines rushing about during the day may make it impossible to sleep undisturbed, even if you are in a totally darkened room. So don't try to sleep during the day rather than at night unless you *have to* because of your job.

Avoid stimulating beverages. In order to make sure that you can take full advantage of regular sleeping hours, you should be careful not to drink coffee, tea, cocoa, or cola drinks in the evening. All these beverages contain nervous system stimulants that can keep you awake at night. It might be all right to have coffee or tea with morning or noon meals, but you'll sleep better if you have milk or juice with your evening meal. Milk has the additional advantage of supplying the calcium you need for calm, relaxed nerves. A glass of warm milk that contains a little honey is an effective bedtime sedative.

Gluttony kills sleep. A light snack at bedtime might actually help you fall asleep by diverting blood from your brain to your stomach. When your stomach is overloaded, however, physical discomfort along with excited nerves may make it impossible to relax, much less sleep.

Salty foods may produce insomnia by stimulating the adrenal glands.

Bed clothes and environment. The type of bed clothing you wear and the environment of your bedroom can play a part in how well you sleep. If the clothing you wear is too coarse, too hot, or too tight, or if your bedroom is too hot or too cold, your senses will be too disturbed to allow your mind to relax. Ideally, the temperature of your bedroom should be about 75 degrees, or just cool enough to permit the use of a light spread or sheet for cover. Bed clothing should not be so tight that it restricts movement or so loose that it tangles. If the temperature of your room is properly adjusted, clothing made from light cotton fabric will be best.

Ventilation is important, but heating or cooling units should not blow directly onto your bed. In the winter, when it's necessary to use heating units, you may have to add moisture to the air to prevent drying of the membranes in your nose. The relative humidity of your bedroom should be about 45 percent. When there is adequate moisture in the air of your home, a temperature of 72 degrees will be comfortable.

Relax your mind and your muscles to sleep better. No matter how carefully you prepare for a good night's sleep, it'll be all for naught if you go to bed with disturbing thoughts on your mind. If you have any problems that must be solved before bedtime, take care of them at least two hours before you begin preparing for bed. Both your mind and your body must be relaxed if you are to get the sleep you need to prolong your life.

HOW TO KEEP A STRAIGHT
SPINE FOR BETTER HEALTH

Everyone knows that bad posture is unhealthy. When the spine slumps, the heart, lungs, and abdominal organs may be dangerously squeezed. Pressure on joints, ligaments, and discs may cause all sorts of aches and pains, some of which may radiate into the legs and arms. In addition to being unhealthy, poor posture is unsightly, and it will give you an aging appearance.

Many of us think that if we maintain good posture in our childhood days we don't need to worry about posture as an adult. The truth is that good posture is just as important for an adult as it is for a child. One reason for this is that as we grow older our bones tend to become softer. If the spine is allowed to slump, softened vertebrae in the upper part of the spine become compressed, causing a permanent hump. This hump is so common among elderly women that it is referred to medically as a "dowager's hump."

After menopause, a hormone deficiency tends to cause loss of calcium in the bones of the spine. When this happens, it doesn't take long for bad posture to produce a permanent hump on the upper back. A few food supplements and a special exercise will help prevent development of the deformity.

Bone-Building Food Supplements

Bone meal with Vitamin D will supply the vitamins and minerals you need for building strong vertebrae. You also need plenty of protein, which is best supplied by chicken, lean meats, and high-protein powders. Just to make sure that you digest your protein and absorb the calcium in your diet, it might be a good idea to take hydrochloric acid tablets with your meals. Discontinue the tablets, however, if they seem to cause digestive disturbances.

Note: If you don't already have osteoporosis or calcium-deficient bones, your bone meal supplements should supply about 800 milligrams of calcium daily. Persons suffering from "soft bones," however, may need as much as 1,500 milligrams daily to get enough calcium to rebuild their bones. Such large amounts are needed because the body absorbs only about 40 percent or less of the amount of calcium taken orally. Bone meal enriched with Vitamin D will automatically supply balanced amounts of all the minerals you need to build bone. If you suffer from kidney stones, you should, of course, talk with your doctor before taking a calcium supplement.

Hormone Therapy for Women

Women who suffer from soft or brittle bones that do not seem to respond to nutritional measures must sometimes be given estrogen (a hormone) to stimulate rebuilding of bone, especially after menopause. Otherwise, progressive deterioration of the vertebrae may eventually result in collapse of the spine. It's best to have an orthopedic specialist prescribe the hormone after studying X-rays of your spine.

**How to Strengthen
Bones with Stress**

Even when the diet is adequate and there is not a hormone deficiency, lack of adequate exercise can result in soft bones. When little or no stress is placed on bones, they lose calcium. Conversely, the more stress there is on your bones the more calcium they store. So while it might be all right to rock in a rocking chair to aid the circulation of blood, you should take some type of regular exercise to stimulate the formation of bone.

Sunlight Strengthens Bones

Sunlight helps strengthen bones by forming Vitamin D on the skin. Remember, however, that sunlight filtered through glass will not supply Vitamin D. So don't attempt to get all the sunlight you need by sitting indoors behind closed windows. Expose your skin to the direct rays of the sun. Be careful, however, not to get a sunburn. Begin with only a few minutes of exposure over a small portion of your body and then gradually increase the exposure.

If you are confined indoors for some reason, you should probably take a little fish liver oil to assure an adequate supply of Vitamin D.

A Spine-Straightening Exercise

Lie on your back with a sofa cushion supporting your upper back. Hold a light weight at arm's length over your chest. About five pounds in each hand, or a single ten-pound weight, will be about right to begin with. Keep your arms locked out straight and lower the weight back over your head to the floor. Inhale deeply as you lower the weight.

This simple exercise will expand your rib cage and stretch your spine out straight. Try to do it at least twice weekly. Whenever possible, do the exercise after a brisk walk so that you'll be breathless enough to benefit from forced deep breathing.

Always remember to "stand tall" and "sit tall." You don't have to worry about observing complicated rules of good posture if you'll simply avoid letting your spine slump.

HOW TO USE MASSAGE
FOR PLEASURE AND FOR
BETTER HEALTH

Massage offers a relaxing and pleasant way to tone muscles and stimulate the circulation of blood. If you're fortunate enough to have a friend or mate who is interested in mutual massage, you can exchange the treatment regularly.

Massage doesn't have to be complicated or strenuous. Basically, all you have to do is mold your hands to the large muscles of the body and rub toward the heart, following the course of the individual muscle. You can use long strokes or short, overlapping strokes, depending upon the size and length of the muscle being massaged. In small areas with short or round muscles, as in the temples and on the chest, circular motions with the hand or the fingertips may be best. The abdomen or a man's chest, for example, is best massaged by keeping the hands in contact with the skin and moving the flesh in a circular motion. (A woman's breasts should *not* be massaged.)

It isn't necessary to hack, vibrate, twist, or use any of the other variations of massage techniques. Simple rubbing or kneading is all that's needed to stimulate the circulation and wake up the body. Just stroke each major muscle group three or four times.

A massage is more effective and more comfortable if it is performed with a lubricant. A little olive oil or mineral oil, for example, should be applied to the skin. You can avoid using too much oil by mixing mineral oil in alcohol. This will enable you to spread the oil in small amounts, so that when the alcohol evaporates it leaves a thin coat of oil on the skin.

When the massage is completed, the oil may be removed with alcohol or rubbed off with a moist cloth. If you suffer from dry skin, just wipe off the excess oil with a dry towel.

HOW TO RELIEVE FATIGUE
CAUSED BY LOW BLOOD SUGAR

If you continue to feel weak, tired, or nervous in spite of all you do to stimulate your body, you might be suffering from hypoglycemia or low blood sugar. A six-hour glucose tolerance test, in which blood samples are tested after drinking a glucose solution, will usually reveal the disorder. The treatment for hypoglycemia is so simple and so effective, however, that anyone suspected of having the disorder can try the treatment without taking a glucose tolerance test.

Nona S. was a school teacher who was constantly complaining about fatigue and inability to concentrate. "Sometimes in the middle of the morning and in the afternoon I get so tired, nervous, and weak that my knees tremble and my legs feel as if they are going to collapse," she said in my office. Nona also told me that she often fell asleep while monitoring study classes, and that she found it difficult to recall facts about subjects she had been teaching for years. She had crying spells that triggered bouts of depression that lasted for days. "I've been to several doctors," she said, "but none of them could find anything wrong with me."

I questioned Nona about her eating habits and learned that she had nothing but coffee for breakfast, that she drank "at least a dozen cups of coffee" each day, and that she frequently had sandwiches for dinner and "TV dinners" for supper. I didn't need to run a blood sugar test to know that Nona was probably suffering from a blood sugar problem. "Rather than go through with a brutal six-hour glucose tolerance test," I told her, "go ahead and try the diet recommended for stabilizing blood sugar. It's a diet that *anyone* can benefit from."

A few weeks later, Nona called to tell me that her fatigue had disappeared and that her mind was once again clear and sharp. If you suffer from any of the symptoms described by Nona, you should try following the same simple suggestions I outlined for her. You'll be glad you did.

**Quit Using Sugar
and White Flour Products**

Most people feel that when they are tired or weak they should eat something sweet for "quick energy." Such snacks do increase energy for awhile. But rapid absorption of sugar and other refined carbohydrates raises the blood sugar level so quickly that the pancreas overreacts by releasing too much insulin. This causes the blood sugar to drop too low three or four hours later. The result is that the brain, muscles, and organs are deprived of the glucose they need for fuel, creating an overpowering mental and physical fatigue. *Everyone* should go easy on sugar and refined carbohydrates.

**Eat High-Protein
Snacks Between Meals**

If symptoms of hypoglycemia persist in spite of eliminating sugar and refined carbohydrates and eating three balanced meals each day (see Life Extender #1), it may be necessary to eat frequent small meals or eat protein snacks between meals. Protein-rich foods such as cottage cheese, baked chicken, peanut butter, or nuts, for example, provide long-lasting energy without stimulating the pancreas. Skim milk, fresh fruit, or unsweetened fruit juice will also supply energy without kicking blood sugar too high.

Remember that most processed or packaged foods contain sugar or refined carbohydrate. If you eat fresh, *natural* foods, it's not likely that you'll have a blood sugar problem. Frequent small meals of natural foods, or high-protein snacks between meals, may even help you reduce excess bodyweight by preventing the hunger that causes you to overeat.

Another Warning About Caffeine

The caffeine in coffee, tea, cocoa, and cola drinks can trigger hypoglycemia by stimulating the adrenal glands, causing the liver to dump too much glucose into the blood. A tired and overly sensitive pancreas may then release too much insulin, resulting in low blood sugar. The lift you get from a cup of coffee, for example, may be followed by a letdown a couple of hours later.

Don't get into the habit of taking coffee or cola breaks. If you feel that you need a pick-me-up beverage between meals, drink milk or juice — or try the Tiger's Milk cocktail recommended under Life Extender #1. The lift you get will be harmless and lasting.

HOW TO COPE
WITH AGING STRESS

It's now well known that repeated and unrelieved stress causes premature aging and disease by flooding the body with hormones that damage blood vessels and organs. Stress also burns great quantities of Vitamin C. When you are suffering from emotional stress, marital problems, insomnia, long working hours, cold weather, fatigue, pain, and other forms of stress, you can benefit from a supplement containing Vitamin C. *The more adrenalin you secrete in tense situations the more Vitamin C you need.*

The B vitamins are also helpful in coping with stress. Yeast and desiccated liver are good sources of all the B vitamins. When your nervous system begins to suffer from prolonged stress, you may need to take a high-potency Vitamin B complex supplement with Vitamin C.

Note: Remember that alcohol destroys B vitamins in the body, and that the nicotine from the smoke of one cigarette can destroy as much as 25 milligrams of Vitamin C in the blood. So no matter what you hear about centenarians who drink and smoke, it's best not to indulge if you want to live as long as you possibly can.

How to Use a Wet-Sheet Pack to Relieve Tension and Nervousness

When stress and tension build to the point where you begin to suffer physically and mentally, a neutral wet-sheet pack will provide immediate relief.

How to apply a wet-sheet pack. All you need for this treatment is a cool, moist sheet and a couple of dry, woolen blankets. Pick a time for the treatment when you have a few extra hours for sleeping. Chances are you'll fall asleep a few minutes after beginning the treatment.

Cover your mattress with a sheet of rubber or plastic, followed by two woolen blankets. Next wring out a sheet in cool water and spread it over the blankets.

Lie down on the sheet and lift your arms while someone folds one-half of the sheet over your body from your armpits to your feet. Then lower your arms while the other half of the sheet is folded over your body from your neck down. Press the sheet down between your thighs and legs to prevent contact between bare skin surfaces. The woolen blankets may then be folded over your body, one side at a time, so that they can be overlapped and tucked under your body for a close fit. If your feet feel cold, they can be warmed with a hot water bottle.

The wet sheet will feel a little cold in the beginning but should feel comfortable after a while. Remember that it's important that you be warm and not hot. When you begin to feel hot, peel back one of the blankets. *If you can maintain a neutral temperature (about 94 degrees), you'll relax and fall asleep.*

Make sure that the blankets are sealed around your neck and feet so that air won't circulate under the moist sheet and chill your body.

After you have been lying relaxed for an hour or so, remove the blankets and the sheet and rub your body with a cold, wet wash cloth for a tonic effect. This should leave you feeling relaxed and refreshed.

If you find that you do not react beneficially to the wet-sheet pack, you may simply take a warm tub bath for relaxation. Some people have such poor circulatory reaction that they cannot recover from the initial chill of a cool, moist sheet.

How to Take a Relaxing Tub Bath

If you use a tub bath to relieve your tension, make sure that the temperature of the water is no higher than 98 degrees Fahrenheit. Water that is too hot (or too cold) will be stimulating rather than relaxing. Fill the tub with water and then adjust the faucet and the overflow so that you can maintain a temperature between 94 and 98 degrees. Lie in the tub and soak in the warm water until your tensions melt away.

Summary

1. Exercise followed by deep breathing will clean out your lungs as well as aid the circulation of blood.
2. Vitamin B_{12} supplied by foods of animal origin, along with wheat germ, brewer's yeast, and green leafy vegetables, will keep your blood rich and healthy.
3. Persons over the age of forty must often take hydrochloric acid tablets to aid in the absorption of iron, Vitamin B_{12}, and calcium.

4. A diet low in animal fat, supplemented with vegetable oil, lecithin, B vitamins, and Vitamin E will help keep your arteries clean and youthful.

5. Regular walking exercises will improve circulation, strengthen your heart, and lower your pulse rate.

6. Leg ache caused by varicose veins can be relieved by elevating the legs, but the legs must be *lowered* to relieve pain caused by hardened arteries.

7. Adequate sleep, a rocking chair, a slant board, good posture, sunlight, and massage are all useful in improving health and delaying the aging process.

8. Brittle bones can result from inactivity as well as from a deficiency in stomach acid, calcium, or Vitamin D.

9. Low blood sugar caused by excessive use of sugar and refined carbohydrates can cause fatigue and other symptoms of aging.

10. Simple massage or a wet-sheet pack applied at home can relieve tension as well as stimulate circulation.

LIFE EXTENDER #5

How to Reverse the Effects of Aging with Home Remedies for Chronic Ailments

As we grow older, the cumulative effects of wear and tear, along with the aging process, result in the development of a variety of chronic ailments. No matter how well you care for your body, or what preventive measures you take, you won't be able to completely avoid certain chronic ailments. Arthritis and hardened arteries, for example, commonly occur among persons past middle age. Fortunately, there are many natural remedies that *you* can use to relieve the symptoms of almost *any* chronic ailment, and these same remedies will help you delay the aging process by improving your health.

Chances are you're already suffering from two or three chronic ailments. Many of us will eventually suffer from *all* the ailments discussed in the next few pages. So be sure to keep this book handy for future reference.

OSTEOARTHRITIS: THE DISEASE OF OLD AGE

When arthritis begins early in life, it may be a serious, crippling form of *rheumatoid arthritis* that should be under

a doctor's care. Arthritis that begins after middle age, however, is usually a chronic, painful, but not often crippling
osteoarthritis. No one knows all the causes of arthritis, and
it's generally believed that there is no cure for arthritis.
There are, however, many home treatment methods that
anyone can use to relieve the symptoms of arthritis, in many
cases preventing stiffness and other crippling effects.

Remember that when any joint pain becomes worse, or
fails to respond to home remedies, you should consult a
physician for more specific diagnosis and treatment. Gout,
infection, and other causes of joint pain may require special
medication for relief of pain.

Moist Heat is the Best
Treatment for Arthritis and Myositis

A fomentation, or simple moist heat, is one of the best
treatments we know of for relieving the symptoms of arthritis, muscular inflammation, and spasm — and the circulatory
effect of such treatment improves the health of joints and
tissues. Best of all, it can be used safely and effectively by
anyone.

Connie E. had long been crippled by arthritis in both
knees. She suffered from constant soreness and stiffness that
periodically flared into painful disability that made it difficult or impossible for her to do her housework. "I've tried
all kinds of drugs and treatments," she said with a note of
discouragement, "but nothing seems to help." When I recommended moist heat applications, Connie replied that she used
a heating pad often but it didn't seem to do much good.
I quickly explained that moist heat was far superior to dry
heat, and that the two cannot be compared. With that, Connie
reluctantly agreed to "go to all the trouble of using moist heat."
On her next visit to my office, she declared that moist heat
applications had proved to be more effective than anything she
had ever tried in treating her arthritis. "Moist heat gives me
more relief than all the expensive treatments I've had — and I
can hardly believe that it doesn't cost me a cent!"

If you suffer from arthritis, you may find that moist heat will give you as much or *more* relief than diathermy treatments in a doctor's office. So don't fail to try it.

The simplest way to apply moist heat is to wring out a towel in hot water and then place it over the painful joint. To conserve heat and moisture, however, and to prolong the effects of the heat, it's best to encase the towels in flannel or wool. Or better yet, instead of using towels, use a flannel material that is about 50 percent wool and 50 percent cotton. The cotton will hold moisture, while the wool holds heat, making a very effective moist heat application. It might also be a good idea to lay a sheet of plastic or rubber over the fomentation to hold in heat and moisture.

Many of my patients report that an insulated heating pad placed over a moist towel provides effective moist heat for one long, continuous application. A hot water bottle wrapped in a moist towel may also be used. Or you may simply use the rays of an infrared bulb to keep the fomentation hot.

Many drug stores sell a "hydrocollater pack" that will hold moist heat for 45 minutes or longer after it has been boiled in water. The pack is simply laid over towels that have been placed over a sore or painful area (especially the back). It may be necessary to use two or three layers of slightly-moist towels under the pack and then remove one or more of the towels as the pack cools.

No matter what type of heat you use, be careful not to burn yourself. *Limit heat treatments to about 20 or 30 minutes,* applied about every two hours. If you do use two or more successive applications of heat, be sure to dry the skin before each application. Water pooled on the skin when a streaming hot pack is applied can result in a bad burn.

Don't ever go to bed with a heating pad and then fall asleep! I've seen many bad burns that have resulted from sleeping with a heating pad, and almost without exception the victim maintains that the pad did not feel hot. Prolonged application of heat that "feels comfortable" may cause tissue damage after several hours.

Note: When application of heat to a painful joint causes an increase in pain, use a cold pack instead of a hot pack. An acutely inflamed joint is sometimes aggravated by heat.

Don't ever use heat over "dead" areas where you cannot distinguish hot from cold.

How to Treat Your Hands, Feet, and Knees with a Paraffin Bath

When arthritis occurs in the hands and feet, simply immersing them in a pan of comfortably hot water (100 to 110 degrees F.) will often provide dramatic relief. A paraffin bath, however, may provide longer-lasting relief by sealing in moist heat. Physical therapists often use paraffin baths in the hospital treatment of arthritic patients. You can use such treatment right in your own home.

How to Prepare a Paraffin Bath

Melt four pounds of ordinary grocery store paraffin in the top of a double boiler and mix in about one-half pint of mineral oil — or simply mix four parts paraffin to one part oil. Paraffin is highly flammable. So be sure not to spill any over an open flame. The more oil you add to the paraffin, the less heat you need to melt the paraffin. Conversely, the smaller the amount of oil added, the hotter the paraffin is when it reaches the melting point. Thus, the heat of a paraffin bath can be controlled by the amount of oil you add. The melting temperature of pure paraffin will be too hot for most people.

The temperature of a mixture of paraffin and mineral oil should be cooled to 125 to 130 degrees Fahrenheit before applying it to your body. If you don't have a bath or candy thermometer to measure the temperature of melted paraffin, let the paraffin cool until the surface congeals. Then test the temperature by inserting a stick of paraffin into the melted paraffin. If the stick melts, the paraffin is too hot to put on your skin. Once you are satisfied that the temperature is not too hot, you can use the paraffin as a dip or as a paint.

How to Use Paraffin as a Dip

A hand or a foot can be dipped into melted paraffin several times to form a wax glove that affords soothing, long-lasting heat. After one quick dip in the hot paraffin, the wax-coated hand or foot can be dipped several times to form a coating about one-quarter of an inch thick. Pause just long enough between dips to allow each new coat to harden. As the coat of wax becomes thicker, the final dips can be prolonged for a greater heating effect. Heat can be preserved by wrapping the wax-coated extremity in oil cloth or a dry towel. Be sure to avoid moving your fingers or toes so that you won't crack the paraffin glove while it's cooling.

Note: For some reason not yet known to medical sleuths, wearing a pair of *stretch gloves* while sleeping tends to eliminate the painful morning stiffness in arthritic hands. The pressure of a pair of tight gloves probably increases warmth and prevents swelling.

How to Paint Joints with Paraffin

You can also use the paraffin treatment on your back, knees, or elbows by painting the paraffin on with a brush. First shave off the hair over the area to be treated — or lubricate the hair with oil — so that you won't pull out the hair when you peel off the paraffin. You may have to wrap an elbow or knee with gauze that can serve as an anchor for painted-on paraffin. Just apply the paraffin with a paint brush until you build up a thick coat.

Paraffin applied to the body will stay warm for 30 minutes or longer. When it cools, peel it off the skin and save it. You can use the same paraffin over and over. You can clean dirty paraffin by heating it in water and then pouring off the water.

Note: Do not apply paraffin or any other form of heat to your feet if you have diabetes or poor circulation. If your feet or ankles are discolored by circulatory deficiency, application of heat might cause tissue damage.

How to Prevent Arthritic Deformities

When joints begin to stiffen from arthritis, it's very important to make sure that you make an effort to maintain a normal range of movement in the affected joints. Move your joints in all directions every day. Exercise just enough to maintain your flexibility, but not so much that you suffer a painful reaction. You'll have to determine from experience how much exercise is best for you.

It's absolutely essential that you develop the habit of sitting and standing erect. Once an arthritic spine stiffens in a slumped position, it tends to become progressively more slumped under the pull of gravity. If you sit a great deal, get up and stretch frequently. Make sure that the mattress you sleep on is firm and smooth. Don't get into the habit of sleeping with a pillow under your knees or with two pillows under your head. If you are confined to bed because of arthritis or illness, lie as straight and as flat as possible.

How to Warm Up Muscles with Liniments

Moist heat stimulates circulation in muscles and joints. Follow that with massage and a heat-producing liniment and you've got a long-lasting treatment for soreness and stiffness. A little oil of wintergreen mixed in mineral oil makes a "hot" massage lubricant. Plain mustard or turpentine can be used in an emergency. Salt, dry mustard, and kerosene are sometimes mixed together and rubbed on the skin. Even horseradish has been mixed in an equal amount of kerosene for use as a liniment. With a little imagination, you can concoct all kinds of liniments. Just be careful not to make them so strong that you blister your skin. Any liniment that produces a little reddening on the skin will relieve deep pain and soreness through a process called counterirritation.

How to Construct a Heat Cabinet

If you have arthritis in all your joints and you want to heat your entire body, you can soak in a tub of hot water — or you can construct a baker made of tin foil and light bulbs. All you have to do is construct a half-circle frame lined with tin foil and evenly-spaced light bulbs. Just make sure that the tin foil is at least 18 inches away from your body on all sides. You can control the heat by using certain size light bulbs or by lighting a certain number of bulbs. Leave each end of the baker open to allow the circulation of air.

Don't lie under the baker longer than half an hour at a time. Put a cold pack on your forehead to make sure that you don't suffer from heat illness. Always follow each heat treatment with a warm shower that's gradually turned down to a cool temperature.

HOW TO RELIEVE LEG AND ARM PAIN CAUSED BY ARTHRITIS

Arm or leg pain is a common complication of spinal arthritis. When bony spurs develop around the vertebrae, they may irritate spinal nerves and cause pain, numbness, tingling, and other symptoms to radiate into an arm or a leg. "Sciatic neuritis," for example, is a leg ache that can often be traced to the back. If the ache reaches below the knee into the foot, a spinal nerve in the lower part of the spine may be irritated or pinched. If the ache is felt on the front of the thigh, the upper lumbar vertebrae may be involved.

Pain on the front of the thigh just above the knee may originate in a hip socket. You can test your hip by sitting down and lifting your foot off the floor (by bending your hip) on the affected side, or by placing the ankle of the affected leg on the knee of the opposite leg. If either of these two maneuvers causes pain in your groin, you may safely assume that something is wrong with your hip. The diagnosis must be made with an X-ray examination.

I have seen many patients with hip trouble that was mistakenly believed to be knee trouble because pain was being referred from the hip to the knee. When I told 72 year old Martin B. that he had hip arthritis, for example, and that there was nothing wrong with his knee, he didn't believe me. "I've been to two different doctors," he argued, "and they both said I had knee trouble." I sent Martin to an orthopedic specialist who confirmed my diagnosis. The point of this little story is that you should never hesitate to seek the opinion of a specialist when pain is persistent or unrelieved. No doctor should ever object to your request to be examined by another doctor.

Leg pain of any kind should always be brought to the attention of a doctor in order to rule out circulatory disorders. Sudden onset of leg pain accompanied by a change in the color or temperature of the leg, for example, may be the result of a blood clot — and that can be very serious if it is not taken care of immediately.

Arm pain should always suggest a heart examination. Most of the time, however, arm pain has a mechanical origin. If it's being caused by a pinched spinal nerve, there may be pain or numbness radiating down the arm into only two or three fingers. Shoulder pain caused by an arthritic spur pinching a spinal nerve is often mistaken for bursitis or tendonitis. When there is something wrong with the shoulder itself, however, movement of the arm will cause shoulder pain.

Once you are satisfied that your leg or arm pain is being caused by spinal arthritis, you might be able to relieve your discomfort by stretching your spine.

Note: When there is burning and tingling in your hands and feet for no apparent reason, try taking Vitamin B_6 (pyridoxin). Women who take birth control pills are often deficient in Vitamin B_6.

How to Stretch Your Neck

Neck, arm, and shoulder pain caused by neck arthritis is so common that just about everyone can benefit from a little neck stretching. You can purchase a "cervical traction" apparatus in any surgical supply store. It usually consists of an overhead pulley and a harness that fits around the head and under the chin. A weight is attached to the loose end of a cord that runs from the harness and over the pulley. A steady pull on the neck relieves pressure on nerves by pulling the bones of the neck apart a little. The traction may be applied while sitting or while lying down, whichever is most convenient for you.

Begin your traction by using about five pounds for 15 minutes. If no ill effects occur, try using ten pounds for several minutes. Be guided by the way you feel. Select the amount of weight that feels best to you. If five pounds relieves your pain, it's not necessary to use a heavier weight. Be careful not to use so much weight, or stay under the traction so long, that you experience an increase in pain or discomfort.

If you don't have a head harness for neck traction, a member of your family can apply traction manually. Just lie on your back on a bed and have someone stretch your neck by pulling on the base of your skull. Your neck should simply be stretched out as far as it will go two or three times.

HOW TO RELIEVE
LOW-BACK NERVE PRESSURE

When leg pain or numbness is the result of a "slipped disc" or an arthritic spur, a little stretch on the lower spine might relieve the symptoms by relieving pressure on nerves. You can stretch your spine at home with a special pelvic harness that can be purchased at any surgical supply store. A weight is attached to the end of a cord that runs from the harness and over a pulley that is fastened to the foot of the bed. You'll need to use about 20 pounds or more for a least half an hour for good results.

You might be able to relieve nerve pain in your legs simply by lying down and draping your legs over the arm of a sofa. If that doesn't help, lie down on your side and roll up into a ball by pulling your knees to your chest. Do so gently, however, and stay well within a range of comfort.

HOW TO CARE FOR BACKACHE AT HOME

There are many causes of backache. If your back aches for no apparent reason, and you do not feel any discomfort when you bend or move about, you might be suffering from kidney trouble or some other abdominal or pelvic disorder that causes backache. If your back trouble is mechanical in nature, that is, if you are sore and stiff and you feel pain when you bend or twist your back, there are several basic treatment methods that you can use at home to relieve your discomfort.

Note: If your backache grows worse after a couple of weeks of self help, or if it lasts longer than six weeks, see your doctor for a checkup — just to make sure that nothing serious is wrong. Backache accompanied by fever is usually the result of an infection, and should be attended by a doctor.

Persons who have had surgery for a malignancy of any kind should suspect a spinal malignancy when there is a persistent backache of unknown origin. Backache that is the result of a malignancy grows progressively worse from day to day and usually hurts more during the night. If your doctor fails to find a cause for your backache, ask him to re-examine you periodically. Spinal malignancy in women who have had breast cancer, for example, may not become evident on X-ray examination for many months after back pain begins. Prostate cancer may also spread to the spine. In fact, spinal cancer almost always occurs secondarily to malignancy somewhere else in the body.

Moist Heat Relieves Backache

Moist heat, such as that described for the treatment of arthritis, is especially beneficial for backache. Towels wrung out in hot water and placed over the back, for example, or simply standing under a hot shower with a heavy stream of water directed over the painful area, will usually afford relief. Any of the heating techniques described earlier in this chapter should be equally effective. I frequently recommend that my patients lay a hot water bottle or an insulated heating pad over moist towels that have been placed directly over the painful area.

Caution: If your heating pad isn't insulated against moisture, you should lay a sheet of rubber or plastic over the towels before applying the pad. Otherwise, you might suffer a painful shock.

**How to Get Pain Relief
with a Poultice or a Plaster**

If you'd like to try a different type of heat treatment on your aching back, a flaxseed poultice or a mustard plaster might be more effective than simple moist heat in relieving pain. Both provide moist heat, but with certain additional benefits.

How to Make a Flaxseed Poultice

To make a flaxseed poultice, boil one cup of flaxseed in one and one-half cups of water until it has a doughy consistency. Then remove the pot from the stove, add one-half teaspoon of soda bicarbonate and beat thoroughly. Spread the mixture about one inch thick between two pieces of warm muslin. Fold the edges of the muslin over to prevent leakage. Lay the poultice over the painful portion of your back.

The poultice should stay warm for 30 to 45 minutes. If you have trouble with dry skin, rub your back with vegetable oil after the poultice has been removed.

How to Make a Mustard Plaster

To make a mustard plaster, mix one part mustard with four to six parts of flour in just enough warm water to make a smooth paste. The moisture in the plaster causes the mustard to release an oil that generates heat by irritating the skin. Remember, however, that if mustard is heated to a temperature above 140 degrees, it won't release the oil.

Spread the mustard mixture about one-fourth of an inch thick between two sheets of warm muslin. Fold the edges of the muslin over to prevent leakage. Then lay the poultice over the painful portion of the back. Lift the plaster every five minutes and examine the skin for redness. Remove the plaster as soon as a definite pickness appears — usually after five to 20 minutes.

Sleep on a Good, Firm Mattress

No matter what type of back trouble you have, a good, firm mattress will help relieve the symptoms. A too-soft, sagging mattress can actually *cause* backache, and it can greatly aggravate a bad back.

If you cannot afford to buy a custom-made or orthopedic mattress, you may place a sheet of plywood between the mattress and the springs, or simply place your mattress on the floor. Essentially, a mattress should be firm enough to keep your spine from sagging, but not so firm that it will not mold itself to the contours of your body. A cotton or felt mattress may be better than an expensive inner-spring mattress.

If you use a board to firm-up an old mattress or to keep a mattress from sagging, use a sheet of plywood that's at least one-half of an inch thick. Cut the plywood so that it will be a little smaller than the mattress and then round the corners so that there won't be any sharp projections.

Persons who suffer from spinal arthritis may find that a bed board will greatly relieve morning soreness and stiffness.

Remember that no matter how young you appear to be, you won't be able to *act* young if your spine is stiff and painful. You can learn more about how to care for your back and spine in my book *Backache: Home Treatment and Prevention* (Parker Publishing Company, West Nyack, New York).

HOW TO RELIEVE MUSCLE SORENESS

It's unfortunately true that the older we become the less active we become. This means that everytime we indulge in a little unaccustomed activity, we experience muscle soreness, but when soreness does occur it can be relieved best by combining muscle contraction with moist heat and massage.

Apply hot, moist towels (wrapped in flannel) over the sore muscles, or stand under a hot shower and let a heavy stream of water run over the affected muscles. Then lightly contract the muscles several times to pump fresh blood through the warmed muscle fibers. Follow this with a little massage using cocoa butter, vegetable oil, or mineral oil as a lubricant. If you really want to give your muscles a glow, mix a little oil of wintergreen with mineral oil for use as a massage lubricant.

Even when your muscles aren't sore, the combined effects of moist heat, muscle contraction, massage, and a warming liniment will help rejuvenate muscles by flushing them with blood and cleaning out waste products.

HOW TO RELIEVE NIGHTLY LEG CRAMPS

When nightly leg cramps occur among young people, we usually think of calcium deficiency. But when they occur among older people, we think of poor circulation *and* calcium deficiency. Since most older people need extra calcium, it's always a good idea to take a calcium supplement — and possibly hydrochloric acid tablets to assure absorption of the calcium. When poor circulation is the cause of leg cramps, there are a few special measures that can be taken to improve circulation and relieve spasm.

How to Flush Leg Arteries with Blood

When leg cramps are the result of poor circulation, the arteries are usually involved. Hardened or clogged arteries, for example, may fail to supply the leg muscles with adequate blood and oxygen when the muscles are relaxed and the body is horizontal. When this happens, leg cramps can often be relieved simply by walking. (See Life Extender #4 for more information about hardened arteries.)

Sitting in a bathtub and rubbing your legs with a hot, wet towel will increase blood flow through leg muscles. Remember, however, that hot applications should not be placed over areas where the circulation is so poor that discoloration is present. You should not massage your legs if they are crippled by venous blood clots.

When the feet and ankles are painful and discolored because of circulatory deficiency, a hot pack placed *over the abdomen* may reflexly increase the circulation enough to relieve cramps. Simply sponging the feet with warm water, or covering the feet with a woolen blanket, may provide adequate heat.

One or two ounces of whiskey or brandy will improve circulation by dilating blood vessels. Niacin and Vitamin E might also be useful in relieving leg cramps caused by poor circulation.

If nightly leg cramps persist because of hardened leg arteries, it might be a good idea to place a brick under the
head posts of your bed so that gravity can aid the flow of
arterial blood into your legs and feet.

Note: When leg pain becomes severe, or if obvious color
or temperature changes occur in a foot or ankle, see your
doctor as soon as possible. Circulatory obstruction caused
by a clot or spasm could lead to loss of a foot if left
unattended.

HOW TO CONTROL YOUR BLOOD PRESSURE

It's well known that high blood pressure tends to shorten
life. Ask your doctor what your blood pressure is the next
time he examines you. If it's higher than "150 over 90," you
should begin taking steps to bring it down.

High blood pressure by itself kills about 60,000 people
each year, and contributes to a million more deaths from
strokes and cardiovascular disease. It is estimated that about
one out of every seven adults has high blood pressure or
hypertension. You can have high blood pressure without any
symptoms whatsoever. So be sure to have your pressure
checked occasionally, even if you don't feel ill. Remember
that blood pressure fluctuates. It should be taken several
times before a diagnosis of hypertension is made.

Unrelieved high blood pressure might eventually damage
the kidneys. In chronic hypertension, for example, the arteries
in the kidneys constrict to reduce the amount of blood flowing
through the kidneys. As a result, the kidneys manufacture too
much renin, which causes the blood pressure to go even higher.
Thus, a vicious cycle develops in which high blood pressure
and kidney damage eventually lead to stroke or failure of the
heart or the kidneys.

Note: If one side of your face should droop suddenly, that
does not necessarily mean that you have had a stroke. Bell's
palsy, which is a form of neuritis, can cause a temporary facial
paralysis.

How to Combat High Blood
Pressure Caused by Hardened Arteries

Hardened arteries commonly contribute to the development of high blood pressure. So the first thing you should do to improve the health of your arteries is observe certain dietary rules. Excessive amounts of sugar and animal fat in the diet, for example, contribute to a build-up of blood fat that clogs and hardens arteries. You need a certain amount of fat in your diet, but you can do without sugar completely.

Turn back to Life Extender #4 and study the dietary measures recommended for improving circulation.

Too much salt in your diet tends to raise blood pressure as well as contribute to hardening of the arteries. Actually, you should try to do without table salt, since natural foods contain all the salt your body needs. Foods that have been processed or preserved often contain sodium additives as well as salt. Anything containing sodium in any form can aggravate high blood pressure.

The water you drink may contain large amounts of sodium. Water that has been softened artificially is so rich in sodium that it should not be used for drinking. "Hard water" that is rich in minerals but low in sodium is best for your health. So while you may use soft water for washing, you should drink *hard* water. If you have high blood pressure and the drinking water in your area is rich in sodium, you can remove the sodium (and other minerals) by distilling the water. If you do distill your water, you should supplement your diet with minerals.

Note: If you eliminate table salt from your diet, be sure to eat seafood for iodine — or take a kelp supplement. Persons living in the region of the Great Lakes or the Rocky Mountains, where the soil is deficient in iodine, cannot depend upon vegetables as a source of iodine. And if they cannot use iodized salt because of high blood pressure, they *must* get their iodine from seafood or from supplements. (An iodine deficiency can result in a goiter or a weight problem.)

How to Lower Blood Pressure with Foods

Persons who already have high blood pressure should eat plenty of fresh fruit. The potassium in fruit helps to counteract the sodium in your diet, and the pectin in the pulp of fruit helps combat hardening of the arteries. Vitamins C and P (rutin and bioflavonoids) found in fruit juice will strengthen blood vessels as well as reduce blood fat.

A low-sodium diet of rice and fruit juice (with a vitamin and mineral supplement) is often effective in lowering blood pressure. Such a diet is too low in protein, however, to follow for more than a few weeks at a time. You *must* have protein to maintain the strength of your bones and muscles. (Persons with *low* blood pressure are often advised to go on a high protein diet.)

Smoking can contribute to high blood pressure. So can obesity or overweight. If you have a weight problem, be sure to study Life Extender #9.

Garlic will sometimes lower blood pressure by dilating blood vessels. You can purchase garlic in tablet form in any health food store.

Remember that emotional stress can raise your blood pressure. If you are constantly being subjected to tension or harassment, you may not be able to reduce your blood pressure until you achieve a relaxed state of mind. Emotional stress can be the cause of a great many ailments. If you can learn to control your mental attitude, you can improve your health and prolong your life.

How to Take Your Own Blood Pressure

If you have trouble with your blood pressure, it might be a good idea to purchase your own blood pressure instrument for use at home. Just wrap the cuff of a sphygmomanometer around your left arm a few inches above the elbow. Hook a stethoscope in your ears and place the disc end against the bend of your arm at the bottom edge of the cuff. As you begin to pump up the cuff, you'll hear the thumping sound of your heart. Continue pumping up the cuff until you can no longer hear the sound. Then slowly release the pressure in the cuff until you again hear the thumping sound. Keep your eyes on the gauge. The location of the needle on the gauge when you hear the first thump will be your systolic pressure. Continue to deflate the cuff slowly. When the thumping sound stops, you'll have your diastolic reading.

It may take a little practice to get an accurate reading of your blood pressure. The procedure is so simple, however, that anyone can do it. Just be careful not to pump the pressure of the cuff any higher than necessary to stop the thumping sound. Don't leave a pumped-up cuff on the arm for more than a few seconds, and don't pump the cuff up more than two or three times during any one attempt to measure blood pressure.

When you discover that your blood pressure is abnormally high, slow down and see your doctor.

HOME CARE FOR VARICOSE VEINS

Very few people who pass the middle age mark in life will escape varicose veins. Failure of the one-way valves in the veins of the legs allows blood to back up in the crippled veins, causing them to become knotty and swollen. Too much sitting and standing, along with the pull of gravity, holds stagnant blood in veins that may eventually become inflamed and clogged. This can lead to cramps, swollen ankles, phlebitis, and leg ulcers.

Lying down with your legs elevated will reduce swollen ankles and drain blood out of swollen veins. Wrapping the feet, ankles, and lower leg with a two- or four-inch elastic bandage will then keep the veins compressed so that they won't collect blood. Walking while the legs are wrapped will increase the effectiveness of muscular contraction in pumping blood through the legs.

For more specific remedies in the care of varicose ulcers, phlebitis, and other circulatory problems, see my book *Doctor Homola's Natural Health Remedies* (Parker Publishing Company, West Nyack, New York).

HOW TO RELIEVE THE
SYMPTOMS OF EMPHYSEMA

If you suffer from breathlessness and a chronic cough, you should be examined for emphysema. After forty years of age, the air sacs of the lungs are often hard and enlarged, making it difficult to empty stale air out of the lungs. If you can't blow out a lighted match held at arm's length in front of your face, you may already have an advanced degree of emphysema. The cough you have may be caused by dry mucus that has accumulated in your bronchial tubes. If so, there are a few simple measures that you can use to "clean out" your lungs.

Rudy P. was only 53 when he started coughing and suffering from breathlessness. A doctor diagnosed his trouble as emphysema and announced that there was no cure for the disease. "Just quit smoking and slow down a little," he advised Rudy.

It's true that there is no cure for emphysema, but there's plenty that you can do to relieve the symptoms. Rudy, for example, was plagued by a chronic cough that proved to be embarrassing as well as irritating. But when he used a few simple home remedies to clean out his lungs, he coughed less in public and he could breathe much better when he played golf and worked in his yard. "My disease may be incurable," Rudy declared, "but I get along much better since I started following your suggestions."

Many incurable diseases, such as arthritis and emphysema, can be tolerated in old age only if they are controlled with self-help measures.

How to Loosen Mucus with Moisture

Inhaling moisturized air will soften the mucus in your lungs so that you can cough it up. This will stop the chronic, dry cough that plagues you day and night.

You can add moisture to the air with a commercial vaporizer or by boiling a pot of water on the stove. You can catch the steam from a boiling pot by draping a towel over your head to form a tent. Inhaling steam in a hot shower is an effective and simple way to loosen mucus. You can purchase a pocket nebulizer that mixes water and air into an aerosol that you can use to moisturize your lungs while you work.

How to Drain Bronchial Mucus with a Special Posture

After you have inhaled moisturized air, pound your chest with your fingertips to break loose stubborn mucus. Lie first on one side and then on the other in order to move the loosened mucus from the smaller tubes into the larger tubes. Then lie across a bed with the upper half of your body hanging over the side of the bed so that both of your forearms are resting on the floor. This upside-down position will drain the mucus from your lungs. Be sure to place a bowl beside your head so that you can collect the mucus for disposal.

How to Open Air Passages with Positive Pressure Breathing

Breathing exercises (such as those described under Life Extender #4) will help overcome the effects of emphysema by strengthening breathing muscles. Exhaling forcefully through a small drinking straw will force expansion of collapsed air passages so that you can empty your lungs without rupturing damaged air sacs. Try using the straw to exhale into a large bottle of water. Make the water boil with bubbles. This will create a beneficial positive pressure in your lungs.

TWELVE HOME REMEDIES FOR HEADACHE

About 90 percent of all headaches are caused by simple tension — that is, by muscle tension that irritates nerves and triggers expansion of blood vessels. This type of headache can usually be relieved by using such measures as moist heat, massage, and traction on the muscles of the neck.

Migraine or "sick headaches" are more severe and more difficult to relieve. There is no known cure for true migraine. If you are a female, however, and you suffer from recurring migraine headache, there's a possibility that the hormonal changes of menopause will result in a complete cure.

If your doctor has ruled out organic disease as a cause of your headaches, and they are not accompanied by fever and other symptoms of illness, you may be able to get relief with simple home remedies.

One of my patients, Pamela T., suffered from such severe, recurring headaches that she was forced to resign from her job as a civil service secretary. A visit to a "headache clinic" failed to uncover a cause for her headaches. A physician prescribed drugs that did little more than relieve the symptoms for a few hours. What Pamela needed was something to *prevent* her headaches. Since she was not suffering from any apparent organic disease, it seemed likely that her headaches were being caused by tension. The muscles on the back of her neck were always tight and sensitive, and she was constantly complaining about insomnia and digestive disturbances. So it was apparent that she was a "nervous type" person.

I gave Pamela a list describing 12 home remedies for headache and suggested that she use those that seemed to help her most. "The first three remedies relieved my headache!" she exclaimed later. "And I've discovered that I can use the same remedies to *prevent* a headache from developing. So I use them practically every day — especially when I feel a headache coming on."

Here are the 12 remedies I outlined for Pamela. Try them a few at a time until you discover which work best for you. Use the first three remedies together whenever possible.

1. Apply a hot, moist towel to the back of your neck to relax muscles and stimulate circulation.
2. Have someone massage the muscles at the base of your skull by supporting your forehead with one hand and encircling the back of your neck with the thumb and forefinger of the other hand. The massaging hand should move the skin over the neck muscles in a circular up-and-down motion.
3. Lie down and have someone gently stretch your neck by pulling on the base of your skull.

4. An ice pack over the forehead or on the front of the neck, combined with a hot foot bath, will sometimes relieve headache by decreasing the flow of blood around the brain.

5. The caffeine in a cup of strong coffee, taken orally or injected into the rectum, will sometimes relieve a throbbing headache by contracting swollen blood vessels.

6. Headaches caused by low blood sugar or a hangover can often be relieved by drinking fruit juice that contains a small amount of honey.

7. A migraine headache can sometimes be aborted by taking an enema when the warning signs appear.

8. Wrapping a tight bandage around the head may relieve headache by compressing swollen blood vessels.

9. Light fingertip pressure on the big arteries of the neck or on swollen temporal or scalp blood vessels for a few seconds at a time might relieve a vascular headache.

10. Headache accompanied by a running nose and a watery eye on the side of the pain may be a histamine headache, making it necessary to remain in an upright position to reduce pressure in sensitive blood vessels.

11. A sinus headache can sometimes be relieved by inhaling steam to loosen mucus and then lying down to permit drainage of sinuses.

12. Rest in a dark room, with your head slightly elevated, will usually minimize symptoms until a migraine headache runs its course.

For more information about the cause and cure of headaches, see my book *A Chiropractor's Treasury of Health Secrets* (Parker Publishing Company, West Nyack, New York).

HOW TO PREVENT AND CONTROL
DIABETES AFTER MIDDLE AGE

After middle age, uncontrolled diabetes, when combined with hardened arteries or poor circulation, can be a serious threat to life and limb. Circulation problems in the feet, for example, can be greatly complicated by high blood sugar. In addition to speeding the development of hardened arteries and blood clots, an excessive amount of sugar in the blood retards the healing of injuries and infections. Most of us know someone who had to have a leg or foot amputated because of a circulatory problem or injury that was complicated by undetected diabetes. It's always a good idea to have your blood sugar checked periodically after middle age.

Fortunately, diabetes that develops after middle age can very often be controlled by diet alone. Even if you do not have diabetes, you should attempt to follow the type of diet recommended for the control of diabetes. Basically, this means that you should *completely eliminate sugar and refined carbohydrates from your diet.* Your diet should consist of such *natural* foods as lean meat, fish, poultry, eggs, fruits, vegetables, milk products, and whole grain cereals. Such foods won't flood your blood with sugar, and they'll supply the vitamins and minerals your body needs to improve the function of your pancreas.

No matter what type of diet you follow, you should remain under the care of a physician if you have diabetes. If you take insulin, it may be possible to reduce the amount of insulin you take — or eliminate it completely — if you follow the correct diet. A periodic blood sugar test by your doctor should be used as a guide in judging the amount of insulin you need.

How to Test for Urine Sugar at Home

Persons suffering from untreated or undetected diabetes often complain of frequent urination, excessive thirst, itching, hunger, weakness, or weight loss caused by a spilling over of sugar into the urine. When blood sugar rises above a certain level, the kidneys eliminate the excess sugar.

You can purchase a "urine-sugar kit" in any drug store for measuring the amount of sugar in your urine. Many diabetics use such kits to measure the effects of the foods they eat. When their urine sugar goes up, they cut back on their sweets and starches — or they see their doctor for an adjustment in their insulin intake.

Although diabetes must always be diagnosed by a blood sugar test, it can often be detected by testing the urine for sugar. So it's a good idea for everyone to use a urine-sugar kit at home. All you have to do is drop a tablet into a mixture of urine and water and watch for color changes.

Summary

1. Natural remedies for chronic ailments that occur after middle age will improve health and prolong life.
2. Simple moist heat is the best treatment for the soreness and stiffness of osteoarthritis.
3. After middle age, it's very important to maintain good standing, sitting, and lying-down postures in order to keep stiff joints and soft bones from developing deformities.
4. Arm or leg pain associated with spinal arthritis can often be relieved by stretching the spine.
5. Any persistent or progressive back pain should be checked for possible malignancy, especially when there is a history of surgery for breast or prostate cancer.
6. Leg cramps at night may be caused by calcium deficiency or hardened arteries and can often be relieved with simple self-help procedures.
7. Don't ever put hot applications on feet that are discolored by a circulatory disorder.
8. When your blood pressure rises above "150 over 90," you should examine your diet and your drinking water.

9. The symptoms of emphysema are best relieved with a home-care routine that "cleans out" your lungs.

10. Chronic headache can often be relieved with any one of the 12 home remedies outlined in this chapter.

LIFE EXTENDER #6

How to Relieve
Body Aches and Pains
Quickly and Easily

Most of the ailments we suffer from after the age of 30 will be chronic in nature. None of us, however, will escape acute injuries and ailments; and if they aren't properly cared for with natural remedies, they may develop into *chronic* ailments. It's no secret that the aging process can be speeded by ailments that cripple the body. Quick and effective attention to certain injuries and ailments will contribute to better health as well as to longer life. Keep this book handy so that you can refer to it when you need a little help in relieving your aches and pains.

HOW TO HANDLE
STRAINS, SPRAINS, AND BRUISES

The use of cold packs and hot packs provides an effective way to relieve pain and speed healing when strains, sprains, and bruises occur. It's essential, however, that you follow certain procedures step by step for best results.

Step 1: Relieve pain and swelling with cold. Whenever you suffer any type of injury that will likely result in painful swelling, you should *apply a cold pack immediately.* Cold will constrict the blood vessels and prevent swelling. Any type of cold application will be all right. I usually recommend that you fill a plastic bag with crushed ice and then wrap it in a moist towel before applying it to the injury. Use the cold for at least 20 minutes every two hours. If the moist cold causes aching or discomfort, try wrapping the bag of ice in a *dry* towel.

Use the cold application off and on for at least 12 hours. Wait 36 to 48 hours before applying heat of any kind. Heat applied to a fresh injury will increase pain and swelling by increasing bleeding. Even if you do not use a cold application, you should still wait a couple of days before applying heat.

If you use cold water for the immersion of an injured hand, elbow, or foot, adjust the temperature of the water to about 50 or 60 degrees. A few ice cubes in a pan of water will maintain a comfortable temperature.

Step 2: Speed healing with heat. After 36 to 48 hours have passed following an injury, you may apply heat to speed healing. Continued use of cold after swelling has stopped would only delay recovery by restricting circulation. Moist heat will speed healing by increasing the flow of blood.

You can make a moist heat application by wrapping a hot water bottle in a moist towel. Or you may direct the rays of an infrared bulb down onto a moist towel applied over the injured muscle or joint. If you use hot water for immersion of an ankle or wrist, adjust the temperature of the water to about 105 degrees Fahrenheit. Heat should be applied for about 20 minutes several times a day.

Note: Whenever the application of heat increases pain, always switch to cold.

Step 3: Pump out swollen tissues with a contrast bath. When an injury is four or five days old, a contrast bath will speed recovery by breaking up clots and flushing out blood vessels. All you have to do is immerse the injured part in comfortably hot water (100 to 110 degrees F.) for about four minutes and then in comfortably cold water (50 to 65 degrees F.) for about one minute. Repeat the cycle several times, beginning and ending with hot water. The hot water will dilate blood vessels, while the cold water will constrict them. This opening and closing of the blood vessels will pump blood through the injured tissues, washing out waste products and debris.

The contrast bath is best applied to the hands, wrists, elbows, feet, and ankles. In other parts of the body, you may simply alternate the use of hot packs and cold packs.

The proper sequence in the use of cold packs, hot packs, and contrast baths will help prevent the formation of adhesions, scar tissue, and calcium deposits. I have seen many cases of chronic disability that could be traced to improper care of an injury. Even if you see a doctor for treatment, the treatment you use *at home* will be the most important in assuring a full recovery.

Note: Acute injuries should always be rested for a few days. But when swelling begins to subside, it's important to begin moving the injured muscles and joints to prevent the formation of adhesions. Procede slowly and progressively and stay well within your tolerance of pain. Gradually increase the strength of contraction and the range of movement.

HOW TO RELIEVE A "NECK CRICK"

Arthur B. woke up one morning with a painful, stiff neck. "There's something wrong with my neck," he complained. "It feels as if someone is sticking me with a knife when I try to turn my head to the right."

An examination revealed that Arthur had a simple muscle spasm. When I explained to him that he had probably pulled a neck muscle in an awkward sleeping posture, he was visibly relieved. "I thought I had something really serious," he confessed.

Actually, neck cricks are fairly common; and while they are quite painful, they are usually nothing to worry about. Most cricks will disappear in four or five days, even if you do nothing for them. If a neck spasm does not release after several days, however, the blood flow through the spastic muscle may be reduced enough to allow the accumulation of lactic acid and other waste products. This can lead to more severe spasm and to chronic inflammation.

Just to make sure that your neck crick gets better rather than worse, apply moist heat to your neck several times a day. This will stimulate blood flow and relax muscles so that waste products can be flushed out of the injured muscle.

Note: If a neck crick lasts longer than a week, see your doctor for a checkup. An arthritic process irritating a joint or a nerve may maintain a spasm long enough to result in muscle shortening or a chronic stiff neck. Cervical traction, such as that described under Life Extender #5, may be helpful in relieving prolonged neck spasm.

HOW TO PREVENT DISABILITY
CAUSED BY BURSITIS AND TENDONITIS

If you suddenly develop a shoulder pain that is aggravated by movement, you may have bursitis or tendonitis. Both can be painful and crippling. *Bursitis* occurs when the lubricating sac around the shoulder joint becomes dry and inflamed. It may occur for no apparent reason, but it most commonly occurs following such activities as painting, scrubbing, or waxing the car. *Tendonitis* is an inflammation of the tendons around the shoulder joint, and is usually the result of a strain.

Prolonged bursitis or tendonitis can "freeze" the shoulder with adhesions or shortened tendons, resulting in permanent disability. So be sure to follow through with the program I've recommended for restoring a painful shoulder to normal.

A Follow-Through Program
for Bursitis and Tendonitis

Relieve acute pain with a cold pack. When bursitis or tendonitis is so acute that the slightest movement causes agonizing pain, a cold pack might be effective in relieving the pain. Wrap a bag of crushed ice in a dry towel and apply it to the shoulder for about half an hour. Repeat the application as often as necessary to relieve the pain.

Support the arm with a sling. An arm sling will often pro-vide blessed relief from acute shoulder pain. You can make a sling or you can purchase one from a drug store. Be sure to adjust the sling so that there is no tension on the tendons of the shoulder. When the pain subsides and you are able to move your arm, discard the sling and begin exercising your shoulder.

Stimulate circulation with moist heat. Apply moist heat to your shoulder as soon as you can do so without increasing the pain. A hot shower, a hot water bottle wrapped in a moist towel, or a simple fomentation, for example, applied about 20 minutes at a time, will flush the shoulder with blood and speed recovery.

Loosen your shoulder by swinging your arm. Whenever you find that you are unable to reach around in back or raise your arm above shoulder level because of pain, there's a simple pendulum exercise that you can do to keep your shoulder from "freezing." Just lean forward and let your arm hang down so that you can swing it back and forth and from side to side. Keep your muscles relaxed so that your arm can swing freely like the pendulum on a grandfather clock.

Lift your arm with a pulley. The sooner you can get your arm above your head the better. Reach as far above your head as you can several times a day. If you can't lift your arm above shoulder level because of stiffness, rig up a pulley that you can use to *pull* your arm overhead. All you have to do is run a line over a pulley so that you can use your good arm to pull up the bad arm. Hoist the arm as far as pain will permit, but try to go a little higher each day. Keep using the pulley until you are able to lift your arm overhead without assistance.

HOW TO RELIEVE
HEMORRHOIDS WITHOUT SURGERY

When Patricia A. first discovered blood on her toilet tissue and in her stool, she was terrified. She delayed seeing her doctor for many months for fear of discovering that she had cancer. She was also reluctant to submit to what she considered a personal and embarrassing examination. As a result, she spent many agonizing months worrying about dying from cancer. She also suffered considerable pain and discomfort, which grew worse as the bleeding increased. When she finally visited a proctologist and learned that she had hemorrhoids, she was greatly relieved. The doctor recommended surgery, which she refused.

When Patricia mentioned to me in the office that she had hemorrhoids, I discovered that she was not doing anything to relieve her symptoms. I recommended a self-help program, which proved to be very effective. "No one ever told me what to do for my hemorrhoids," she said later. "Since I've been helping myself, I have very little trouble — and I certainly don't need any surgery!"

Hemorrhoids or "piles" are extremely common after middle age. Actually, hemorrhoids are nothing more than varicose veins in the rectal or anal area. They may be caused by pregnancy, overweight, chronic coughing, toilet straining, exertion during breath holding, and other conditions and activities that increase pressure in the rectal veins. When hemorrhoids become large or obstructed, they may bulge through the anus, become inflamed, bleed, cause pain on bowel movements, or itch severely. They most often cause trouble after straining to empty the bowels or after excessive rubbing of the anal area with toilet tissue.

Properly cared for, an acute attack of hemorrhoids tends to subside after several days. Unless bleeding is severe enough to cause anemia, or the hemorrhoids are large enough to obstruct the anal area or cause intolerable pain, surgery is rarely needed. Once it has been established that you have bleeding hemorrhoids, you should not be alarmed by occasional bleeding.

Note: Blood from the stomach or small intestines will result in a black, tar-like stool. Blood from bleeding hemorrhoids is always bright red.

How to Keep Your Hemorrhoids Under Control

When you visit the toilet for a bowel movement, don't sit on the toilet any longer than necessary — *and don't strain.*

Attempts to forcefully evacuate the lower bowel will cause the rectal veins to swell with blood, resulting in bleeding or inflammation. Be sure to study Life Extender #7 for tips on how to avoid constipation. It's almost impossible to keep hemorrhoids under control if you allow yourself to become constipated.

You can lubricate hemorrhoids and soften your stool by injecting a little olive oil or mineral oil into your rectum just before a bowel movement. Mineral oil taken orally will also lubricate the lower bowel, since the oil passes through the digestive tract unabsorbed. Oral use of mineral oil, however, will result in elimination of fat-soluble vitamins. So I usually recommend rectal injection of oil with a syringe — either before retiring at night or just before a morning bowel movement.

After each bowel movement, clean the anal area by patting it with moist tissue paper or cotton. Or wash the anal area with a sponge filled with cold water and then pat it dry with absorbent cotton. A medicated powder may then be applied to prevent irritating dampness. It may occasionally be necessary to rub a little olive oil on external hemorrhoids to relieve painful friction.

Note: Internal hemorrhoids can be cleaned by using a syringe to inject cold water into the rectum. The water is then expelled, just as you would do when you take an enema.

How to Replace Protruding Hemorrhoids

Internal hemorrhoids that protrude through the anus can usually be pushed back into the rectum. First apply a cold compress to shrink the hemorrhoids. Then apply a little olive oil or mineral oil for lubrication. Lie on your side, or get down on your elbows and knees, and use your fingers to push the swollen veins back through your anus.

How to Relieve the Pain of Hemorrhoids

Moist heat applied to the anal area will very often relieve the pain and itching of external hemorrhoids. You may apply hot, wet towels or pads of gauze to the anus, or you may simply sit in a pan of hot water.

An *anal steam bath* provides an effective way to apply steam and medication simultaneously. Cut a six-inch hole in a wide plank and place it over a bucket that contains steaming hot water. Put in a few drops of turpentine, camphor, vegetable oil, or any other medication you want to use. Sit over the hole in the plank so that steam reaches the anal area. After about half an hour of sitting on the bucket, pat the hemorrhoids dry with gauze or a soft towel.

DIETARY HINTS FOR CONTROLLING GOUT

If you should suddenly develop a severe, throbbing pain in your big toe, foot, knee, elbow, or wrist, you may have gout. This means that uric acid crystals may be accumulating in the joints of your body. A blood uric acid test performed by your doctor will tell whether you have gout or not.

Only about five percent of gouty patients are female, and most of these have gone through the menopause. If you develop gout for the first time after the age of 30, it's not likely to be as severe as that beginning earlier in life, and you may be able to control it with diet. Perry J., for example, had his first attack of gout at the age of 49. A blood test confirmed my suspicion that his swollen, throbbing wrist was the result of gouty arthritis. When I learned that Perry's favorite foods were steak and chili with red peppers and beans, I suggested that he try a few dietary measures before resorting to the use of drugs. That was five years ago. To this day, Perry has not had another attack of gout.

A Dietary Program for Gout

Much of the uric acid that accumulates in the blood may come from a breakdown of body protein. Some comes from purine-rich protein foods such as sweetbreads (animal pancreas or thymus), sardines, anchovies, kidneys, liver, brain, meat, meat extracts, gravies, fish, game, fowl, beans, and lentils. Spices, condiments, and alcoholic beverages are also rich in purine.

Beverages containing caffeine, such as coffee, tea, cocoa,

and cola drinks form purine in the body. So it may be necessary to be careful about what you eat and drink.

Use of penicillin, insulin, or diuretics may trigger attacks of gout in susceptible persons.

I usually advise my gouty patients to get most of their protein from milk and milk products, eggs, cheese, cottage cheese, gelatin, nuts, seeds, and protein supplements. Wheat products should be avoided. Corn bread can replace wheat bread. Grits can replace whole grain cereals. A large part of the diet should be made up of fruits and vegetables. Plenty of liquids — up to three quarts a day — will help the kidneys eliminate uric acid and cut down on the formation of kidney stones. Fruit and vegetable juices will also help prevent the formation of uric acid stones by alkalizing the urine.

Obesity or overweight tends to raise blood uric acid. Remember, however, that too rapid a weight loss may trigger gouty attacks by breaking down nucleic acids in tissue cells. For this reason, you should avoid "crash diets" that result in the loss of more than a few pounds a week. If you need to lose weight, turn to Life Extender #9 and try my natural foods reducing diet.

Additional Facts About Gout

Most attacks of gout will occur in the foot, usually in the big toe. Shoes that are too tight may trigger attacks of gout in susceptible persons. So make sure that your shoes are properly fitted.

When the big toe is swollen, dark red, and throbbing with an attack of gout, even the weight of a bed sheet on the toe can be intolerable. When this is the case, and you cannot sleep with your foot uncovered, you can construct a light, wooden frame to place over your foot so the bed covers won't rest against the painful toe.

An attack of gout will usually subside in a few days, but it will recur if the uric acid level of the blood remains high. Remember that there is no cure for gout. Once the disease develops, you must either reduce your intake of protein foods that contain purine or take medication to relieve gouty attacks. Some patients need only to restrict their intake of organ meats. Others have to restrict meats, poultry, fish, and beans.

Note: If symptoms of gout occur in spite of a carefully regulated diet, it may be necessary to take special medication to aid in the elimination of uric acid produced in the body.

FIRST AID FOR SHINGLES

The sudden eruption of a chain of painful blisters on the skin is usually shingles, caused by virus infection of a nerve trunk. The blisters look very much like fever blisters and are caused by a similar virus. Shingles is most common in persons over 50 years of age.

The blisters most often appear on one side of the back and chest. Many people believe that death will occur if a chain of blisters reaches around the body. That's just an old wives tale that has no basis in fact. So don't worry if shingles encircles your chest or abdomen.

Actually, other than being extremely painful, shingles usually isn't serious, and it begins a self-healing process after five or six days. Shingles can leave scars, however, and in elderly persons there may be persistent pain for months and years after the blisters disappear. Fortunately, one attack of shingles usually provides immunity to the virus that causes the disease. So once you've had shingles, it's not likely that you'll have it again.

There is no known cure for shingles. It simply runs its course. It might be a good idea, however, to take high-potency B complex vitamins. Oatmeal water or cornstarch solutions (see Life Extender #2) applied over the blisters might be soothing. Moist, cool compresses wrung out in water containing sodium bicarbonate would be worth trying for relief of pain.

HOW TO AVOID PERMANENT PARALYSIS IN BELL'S PALSY

You may never have Bell's palsy. But if one side of your face ever sags with what appears to be a sudden paralysis, it might be Bell's palsy rather than a stroke. If so, the paralysis will usually disappear in a few weeks. There are, however, a few things that you can do to relieve discomfort and speed recovery. Wearing an eye patch over the affected eye, for example, will keep the eyelid closed and prevent dryness and irritation of the eyeball. Moist heat and massage applied to the affected facial muscles will help maintain their tone. You might even want to tape up the sagging side of your face for cosmetic reasons. Large doses of B complex vitamins will speed recovery of the inflamed nerve.

HOW TO COPE WITH
THE PAIN OF TIC DOULOUREUX

In Bell's palsy, paralysis occurs without pain. In tic douloureux, or trigeminal neuralgia, severe pain occurs on one side of the face without paralysis. It occurs most commonly after 50 years of age and has no known cause. Stabbing, lightning-like pains that last for a minute or two occur periodically, often triggered by exposure to cold, washing the face, talking, eating, or drinking. Victims often find that they must avoid cold water or cold drinks in order to avoid the pain.

Tic douloureux is so painful that it may be necessary for a physician to prescribe special drugs to withstand recurring attacks. If the attacks become increasingly more frequent and severe, doctors sometimes recommend that the nerve be cut.

HOW TO SPEED
RECOVERY FROM A COMMON COLD

Cold infections occur among all ages, but they can be more serious among older people. When resistance is low because of poor health, a common cold can lead to pneumonia, bronchitis, sinus infections, and other serious ailments. And the older you are the more serious the infection may be. When a 20 year old person develops pneumonia, for example, his chances of dying are only about two in 100,000. But when an 85 year old person comes down with pneumonia, his chances of dying from the infection are about 1,000 in 100,000.

There is still no known cure for a common cold. In a healthy person, a cold runs a course of about seven days. There is something that you can do to increase your resistance against cold infection, however, and there are measures that you can take to speed recovery, relieve symptoms, and prevent complications. You may even be able to *prevent* a cold by taking certain steps to combat cold germs.

Vitamin C, Garlic, and Other Remedies

I usually recommend that everyone take about 1,000 milligrams of natural Vitamin C daily during the cold season to help maintain resistance against cold germs. When a cold begins to develop, however, the dosage of Vitamin C should be increased to about 500 milligrams every hour for several hours. It's better to take Vitamin C periodically throughout the day — at least every four hours — than to take one large dose. Taking all your Vitamin C at one time will force your kidneys to eliminate much of the vitamin.

Garlic is a potent germicide that may be helpful in killing cold germs. Try to eat a little garlic during the cold season.

Inhaling steam that contains a little vinegar may help kill germs in the throat. All you have to do is put a spoonful of vinegar into a pot of boiling water and then inhale the steam. (The secretions of the nose are normally slightly acid. When a cold first begins, however, the nose and throat become dry and alkaline, allowing invasion by germs.)

Plenty of fruit juices and water will replace fluids lost through the membranes of the nose as well as aid in flushing out cold germs. Drink plenty of liquids during the early stages of a cold.

Make sure that the relative humidity in your home is at least 40 percent. Cold germs thrive in dry nasal passages. If necessary, you can add a commercial humidifier to your central heating unit — or you can place a pot of water on top of a stove or heater.

Don't let your home get too hot. Dashing out into winter cold from a hot room isn't good for anyone. Sudden and extreme changes in temperature can weaken mucous membranes and set the stage for cold infection or a sore throat.

When a cold passes the watery stage and the nose becomes clogged with thick mucus, inhale a little steam to loosen the mucus before blowing your nose. Blowing your nose too forcefully might force germs into your sinuses or your inner ear and result in a painful infection. (Smelling onion or garlic will often open a stuffy nose.)

Get plenty of rest. Remember that if a cold lasts too long, it will lower your resistance and lead to more serious infections.

HOW TO HELP NATURE HEAL FRACTURES

You learned with Life Extender #4 that you must have adequate amounts of calcium, phosphorus, Vitamin D, magnesium, and protein to maintain strong bones. When you fracture a bone, you need increased amounts of these essential food elements to assure rapid and solid healing. I usually recommend bone meal tablets (with Vitamin D), along with a little daily exposure to sunlight. Bone meal powder and powdered skim milk can be added to soups, meat loaf, homemade bread, and other foods for additional minerals and protein. A balanced diet is, of course, essential, no matter what type of supplements you take.

Stay as active as possible while recovering from a fracture. If you are not confined to bed, go outdoors and use your muscles. If a splint or cast prevents movement of joints, contract or tense your muscles isometrically. Bones become weak and thin when they are not subjected to stress. When a fracture heals, early use of muscles will strengthen the new bone.

If a fracture is slow in healing, or if your bones break easily in spite of an adequate supply of minerals, you may not be absorbing the calcium or Vitamin D you need. A deficiency in stomach acid, for example, can prevent absorption of calcium. (This can be corrected by taking hydrochloric acid tablets with your meals.) Excessive use of alkalizers or antacids can prevent absorption of calcium by neutralizing stomach acid. Gall bladder trouble can interfere with absorption of Vitamin D. (Tablets containing ox bile might be helpful in the digestion of fats containing Vitamin D.)

Don't let your bones get weak from inactivity or dietary deficiency. Many elderly people have such weak bones that fractures occur spontaneously. A hip fracture, for example, may occur while walking, causing a fall that is mistakenly believed to be the cause of the fracture. I've seen many rib and spinal fractures that have occurred as a result of such simple stresses as sneezing or moving furniture.

HOW TO HANDLE A HERNIA

No matter how physically fit you might have been in your younger days, you may be subject to hernia after middle age if you allow your abdomen to become fat and flabby. Most hernias occur in the groin area where muscular rings allow blood vessels, nerves, and other structures to pass from the abdomen into the thighs and genitals. When the muscles around these rings become weak and pressures develop from a fat, sagging abdomen, the rings may stretch enough to allow a portion of the intestinal tract to bulge through. This results in a soft, bulging mass in the groin.

The best treatment for hernia is prevention; that is, keeping the muscles of the abdomen lean and well developed. Once a hernia develops, it can never be completely cured. It may be possible to control or reverse its development, however, by reducing your bodyweight and developing your abdominal muscles.

When a hernia is massive enough to cause a large bulge, it can often be manipulated back through the opening while you are lying relaxed on a slant board. A truss may then be worn to keep the opening closed.

Note: Always remember to exhale while straining or while contracting your abdominal muscles during sit-up exercises. Holding your breath while you are exercising, while lifting a heavy object, or while straining to empty your bowels can create enough pressure inside your abdomen to push your intestinal tract through a weak or enlarged femoral or inguinal ring.

HOW TO AVOID SURGERY
FOR A DIAPHRAGMATIC HERNIA

A diaphragmatic hernia occurs when a portion of the stomach bulges through an opening in the diaphragm (the big, flat muscle that separates the chest cavity from the abdominal cavity). Food and gas trapped in the portion of the stomach above the diaphragm (in the chest) may cause chest pain, spasm, belching, and sometimes hiccups.

Wilhelm V. thought he had heart trouble when he began to experience chest pain after eating. "I have a pain in the center of my chest after eating," he said, pointing to his breastbone. "And it gets so bad sometimes that I can't lie down." An X-ray examination revealed a diaphragmatic hernia. Wilhelm was able to relieve his discomfort and avoid surgery by following five simple suggestions. "Now that I know what causes the pain," he said with obvious confidence, "I can avoid it completely."

If you have any of the symptoms of a diaphragmatic hernia, try the five suggestions I've numbered below. Chances are they'll do as much for you as they did for Wilhelm.

**Five Tips for Relieving the
Symptoms of Diaphragmatic Hernia**

1. *Avoid overeating.* If your stomach is overloaded, food trapped above the diaphragm may trigger painful spasm. Frequent, small meals are better than two or three large meals.

2. *Don't lie down after eating.* If you'll remain in a sitting position after each meal, the top portion of your stomach (above your diaphragm) will remain empty.

3. *Avoid spicy foods* that might irritate the stomach if they are trapped above the diaphragm. (Chronic irritation of the stomach can lead to stomach ulcers as well as cause painful spasm.)

4. If you're overweight, *reduce your bodyweight* so that your hernia won't be aggravated by excessive abdominal pressure.

5. When symptoms of a diaphragmatic hernia persist after eating, it may be necessary to elevate the head of your bed in order to sleep comfortably. You can do this by placing eight-inch blocks under both head posts. It may occasionally be necessary to sleep in a sitting position until the stomach can empty itself.

HOW TO REMOVE EAR WAX

An excessive amount of wax in the ear canal can cause earache, deafness, ringing in the ears, and dizziness. It might even trigger a nerve reflex that results in chronic coughing.

If your ears become plugged with ear wax, don't try to wash them out with water. A little warm olive oil or glycerine placed in your ears with a medicine dropper will soften the plugs of wax so that they can be drained. (Warm oil can also be used to ease earache and float out insects and other particles.)

After the oil and wax has been drained from your ear, warm water from an ear syringe can be used to wash out remaining debris. Always tilt your head to one side to drain water or oil from your ear. A cotton bud or a Q-tip can be used to dry the ear canal.

Remember that water trapped in the ear can contribute to the growth of ear fungus. If you develop pain or soreness in an ear canal, see an ear specialist for an examination.

HOW TO CONTROL PSORIASIS

The cause of psoriasis is not known, and there is no specific cure. If an effort is made to control the disease, however, it can be kept from spreading or growing worse. "I still have psoriasis," reported Earnestine W. after treating her skin with home remedies, "but it's much better, and there are times when it's hardly noticeable."

If you develop any red patches on your skin that are covered with shiny scales, follow these suggestions:

1. Bathe your skin each day with mild soap and water. Use a soft skin brush to scrub away the scales.

2. Expose your skin to a few minutes of sunlight or ultra-violet rays two or three times a week.

3. Use cold-pressed vegetable oil on a daily green salad to assure an adequate supply of the essential fatty acids. Take a supplement containing Vitamin B complex, lecithin, and 25,000 units of Vitamin A each day.

4. Occasionally rub the diseased skin with wheat germ oil.

5. Boil meats, fish, and poultry for 10 minutes and discard the water before roasting, broiling, or frying. This will eliminate taurine, a non-essential amino acid believed to contribute to the development of psoriasis. (Soybeans are rich in protein but low in taurine.)

6. Reduce your intake of eggs and animal fat and avoid processed foods containing saturated fat. Remember that margarine or hydrogenated vegetable oil is a saturated fat. So is coconut oil.

HOW TO PREVENT BED SORES

Bed sores occur when prolonged bed rest in one position interferes with the circulation of blood by putting pressure on prominent bony areas. If you must remain in bed a long time because of injury or illness, follow these procedures to prevent bed sores:

1. Sleep on a foam rubber mattress — or pad your mattress with a layer of foam rubber.

2. Make sure that there are no wrinkles in the sheet covering your mattress.

3. Change your position in bed as often as possible — at least every three or four hours. If you must lie on your back, a pillow under your knees and calves will relieve pressure on the back of your heels.

4. Dry your skin thoroughly after each bath.

5. Have someone massage your body with alcohol each day to toughen your skin and stimulate circulation.

DIETARY SUPPLEMENTS FOR NERVOUS TREMORS

If you develop a nervous tremor, supplement your diet with magnesium, Vitamin B complex, and pyridoxine (Vitamin B_6). "It has been my experience," says Adelle Davis in *Let's Get Well,* "that Vitamin B$_6$ and magnesium alleviate tics and tremors quickly or not at all."

Some nutritionists report that Parkinson's disease will respond to Vitamin B$_6$ in doses of 10 to 100 milligrams if accompanied by magnesium and *all* the B vitamins.

Summary

1. Always apply cold to fresh strains, sprains, and bruises. Wait 36 to 48 hours before using heat.
2. Neck "cricks" will usually subside after three or four days if moist heat is applied to the neck three or four times a day.
3. When bursitis or tendonitis develops in the shoulder, a special procedure must be followed to keep the shoulder from "freezing."
4. Injecting olive oil into the rectum will lubricate painful hemorrhoids and aid bowel movements.
5. Gout can sometimes be controlled by restricting use of meats, animal organs, and other foods that are rich in purine.
6. Nerve conditions such as Bell's palsy and shingles can be cared for successfully with simple home remedies.
7. Proper care for a common cold will prevent such serious complications as bronchitis or pneumonia.
8. Bones can be strengthened and the healing of fractures speeded with special dietary supplements, sunlight, and controlled exercise.
9. Abdominal hernia and diaphragmatic hernia can be controlled with special home-care procedures.
10. You'll find many tips in this chapter on how to care for such conditions as clogged ears, psoriasis, and nervous tremors.

   Remember that proper home care for "minor" ailments can prevent the development of *chronic* ailments.

LIFE EXTENDER #7

How to Flush Out
Poisons that Cause Aging

Proper elimination of waste by the body is essential in maintaining good health for a long life. Many people pay close attention to what they eat and then ignore the more unpleasant functions of elimination. Fortunately, the lungs and the skin automatically eliminate much of the metabolic wastes of the body — and they do so in spite of an individual's ignorance of his body. You know from reading other portions of this book, however, that failure to maintain good health can result in disease of the lungs and the skin, thus interfering with elimination. So it's very important to observe *all* the basic rules for building good health.

Kidney function can be aided by a good diet and by special dietary measures. In some cases, a short fast with an increased intake of fluids gives tissue cells a better opportunity to dump accumulated waste products into the blood stream for elimination through the lungs, kidneys, and skin.

The bowels are concerned primarily with elimination of the waste products of digestion. The bowels also work automatically, but how well they function is determined largely by the eating and toilet habits of the individual. There are many things that you can do to improve the function of your bowels, your kidneys, and your skin.

HOW TO IMPROVE ELIMINATION
BY CORRECTING CONSTIPATION

Many people believe that it is essential to have a bowel movement every day. Most people do have at least one bowel movement each day, but there are many people for whom a movement every other day or even every third day is normal. Even if you are accustomed to emptying your bowels every day, no harm will result if you miss a couple of days. Emotional stress, a change in diet or daily routine, traveling, loss of sleep, a back injury, and other disturbing influences can temporarily halt evacuation of the bowels.

Clyde G. complained of constipation the second day after he suffered a back injury. "My bowels haven't moved in two days," he complained with a note of panic. "Can you recommend a good laxative?" Clyde obviously thought that something terrible would happen if his bowels didn't move every day. I advised him to wait two more days and then take an enema if his bowels didn't move. On the morning of the fourth day, he had a normal movement. Had Clyde taken a laxative, he would have had a difficult time getting his bowels back on a regular schedule.

Whenever your bowels fail to move on schedule, don't panic and take a laxative. Chances are they'll move after a couple of days if you'll continue to visit the toilet regularly. If you are truly constipated, your stools will be small, hard, and often in the shape of marbles. It is possible to be constipated and still have a daily bowel movement. Someone who is *not* constipated may pass a complete, normally-formed stool only once every two or three days. So the frequency of bowel movement has little to do with constipation.

Visit the Toilet Regularly

A daily bowel movement is best for most people. You should visit the toilet every day just to make sure that you don't "hold back" your bowels. Set up a regular schedule for visiting the toilet. *Visit the toilet at the same time each day.* Once your bowels have been trained to empty at a certain time, they'll empty with little or no effort. You should never ignore an urge to empty your bowels, however, no matter when it comes. If you consistently fail to visit the toilet when your bowels are ready to empty, the urge may disappear and not return. This may allow the contents of the lower bowel to become dry and impacted, resulting in severe constipation.

Failure to visit the toilet on a regular schedule is probably one of the most common causes of constipation.

Don't Use Commercial Laxatives

When the intestinal tract has been emptied by a commercial laxative, it may be three or four days before the lower bowel needs to empty again. Most laxative users, however, grow impatient after a few days and take another laxative. The bowels soon become accustomed to emptying only when they are stimulated artificially, resulting in the worst kind of constipation. Persons who take laxatives regularly may actually force the intestinal tract to eliminate partially-digested food, depriving the body of the nutrients it needs to be healthy and youthful.

Actually, you should never have to take a commercial laxative. If you eat the right kinds of foods and visit the toilet regularly, your bowels will take care of themselves.

Natural Laxatives Are Best

When constipation does occur, foods and beverages may be your best laxatives. A little lemon juice in hot water, for example, taken before breakfast, will often trigger a bowel movement. Dried prunes soaked overnight in hot water containing lemon juice and honey, taken an hour before breakfast, has proved to be an effective laxative for many people.

Fresh and dried fruits have a laxative effect on most people. A large batch of almost any kind of fruit, eaten in the evening, will help stimulate a morning bowel movement.

Bran provided by whole grain cereals and bread helps stimulate the bowels, but too much bran may be harmful. Pure bran cereals, for example, may fill the lower bowel with a tightly-packed mass that *contributes* to constipation. Bran does not hold moisture, and when a large amount has accumulated in the colon it tends to become dry and hard like sawdust. You can get all the bran you need from whole-grain cereals and breads. So go easy on pure bran cereals.

The cellulose provided by fruits and vegetables leaves a straw-like residue that holds moisture and encourages the growth of helpful bacteria. When there is adequate cellulose in your diet, plenty of drinking water and fruit juices will keep your stools moist and passable.

REFINED CARBOHYDRATES CAUSE DIVERTICULITIS AND COLON CANCER

There are several good reasons why you should avoid refined or processed foods. In addition to clogging your bowels with sticky, constipating waste, an excessive amount of refined foods in the diet can contribute to the development of diverticulitis and colon cancer! When the colon is clogged by the sticky residue of refined carbohydrates, for example, the colon wall is stretched and placed under pressure. Contraction of the colon in attempts to evacuate the waste produces small stretched-out pouches called diverticula. When these pouches become inflamed or clogged with waste, diverticulitis results, causing abdominal pain, diarrhea, and cramps that may be alternated with constipation.

Worst of all, when the colon is filled with the slow-moving wastes of refined carbohydrates, bacterial changes in the colon produce chemicals that may trigger malignant growths. It's significant to note that constipation is extremely common in the United States where refined foods are commonly used and where colon cancer is the second most common cause of death from cancer.

All of this can be avoided by eating natural foods with plenty of fruits and vegetables.

Special Supplements for Cleaner Bowels

If you must go on a low-residue diet for some reason, and you're unable to eat fruits and vegetables, you should supplement your diet with agar or psyllium seed extract. These indigestible products retain water and provide the bulk you need for a moist, well-formed stool. As soon as possible, however, you should resume a normal diet that includes fruits and vegetables. You need all the cellulose you can get to sweep your bowels clean. You'll learn more about how to improve your digestion with Life Extender #8.

How to Empty a Clogged Rectum

Whenever constipation fails to respond to the laxative effects of natural foods, don't attempt to empty your bowels by straining. This might cause hemorrhoids or result in a painful tear at the bowel opening. In some cases, you may be able to relieve constipation simply by inserting your finger into your rectum to breakup a hardened mass. Injecting a cup of olive oil into your rectum at bedtime will soften and lubricate rectal impactions for a morning evacuation. A "quickie enema" with a disposable enema kit, taken during regular toilet hours, will help restore regularity.

How to Take an Enema

Enemas are so safe and so simple that anyone can take them — or give them. Attach an enema tip (with tubing) to a hot water bottle and then fill the bottle with a quart of warm water. A special clamp on the tubing will enable you to control the flow of water.

Hang the water-filled bottle on a wall so that it will be 12 to 18 inches above your buttocks when you get into a position for the enema. Lie on your side with the knee of your upper leg pulled up toward your chest. Release the clamp and run a little water through the tubing to expel the air. Then lubricate the enema tip and insert it three or four inches into your rectum — never more than four inches.

Release the clamp and allow the water to run slowly into your bowel. If cramping or discomfort occurs, stop the flow of water until the discomfort subsides. When the enema bag has been emptied, try to hold the water in your bowel long enough to soften the hardened waste. Then sit on the toilet for a bowel movement.

HOW TO COPE WITH RECTOCELE

Women who suffer from rectocele should be especially careful to avoid constipation. Rectocele occurs when a weak or stretched vaginal wall allows the rectum to bulge forward into the vagina. When the lower bowel is clogged and overloaded, the bulge into the vagina may cause considerable discomfort. Straining to empty the bowels will, of course, increase the size of the bulge.

Constipation can be prevented or relieved by observing the simple rules outlined earlier in this chapter. Squatting down to have a bowel movement will relieve pressure in a rectocele by forcing the bowel to empty toward the back rather than toward the vagina. Or you may simply place both feet on a low foot stool (8 to 12 inches high) while sitting on the toilet, so that your thighs are flexed against your abdomen.

HOW TO RELIEVE GAS PAINS

Gas pains that accompany constipation can often be relieved with simple home remedies. You should first try to get rid of the gas by getting down on your knees and elbows so that the gas will rise to the rectum where it can be expelled. If that doesn't work, an enema made up of one quart of water containing two teaspoons of oil of peppermint might do the trick. Or you may simply drink a cup of hot water containing one drop of oil of peppermint.

A hot pack placed over your abdomen will often relieve acute gas pains. But you must first make sure that you don't have an inflamed or infected appendix. Always see your doctor when abdominal pains are accompanied by fever.

Taking baking soda or an alkalizer to relieve gas pains may only cause *more* gas when the alkali reacts with stomach acid. Health food stores sell charcoal tablets that are reported to be helpful in overcoming gas pains.

Swallowing air while eating, drinking, or chewing is a common cause of "gas." Try to keep your mouth closed while you are chewing or swallowing. Gas or air in the stomach can be belched up, but when it becomes trapped in the intestinal tract it must be passed through the rectum as "flatulence."

Foods such as beans, green salads, cucumbers, onions, cabbage, and milk commonly cause gas. If you think that something you're eating is producing gas in your intestine, eliminate the suspected foods from your diet for a few days and see if any improvement occurs.

You'll learn more about what causes intestinal flatulence when you reach Life Extender #8. Remember that any kind of intestinal disturbance may mean that you aren't absorbing all the nutrients you need to live a long, healthy life. So the more you can learn about digestion and elimination, the better.

HOW TO IMPROVE THE
FUNCTION OF YOUR KIDNEYS

Everyone knows that the kidneys absorb wastes from the blood to form urine. Normal, healthy kidneys can handle the toxins unloaded by the blood, but you can protect your kidneys and prevent an overload by being careful about what you eat. Excessive use of sugar, for example, may force the kidneys to eliminate glucose that is "spilled over" from the blood. Diets made up entirely of protein may overwork the kidneys with the waste products of protein metabolism. Some processed foods contain chemical additives that may place an abnormal strain on the kidneys. And so on.

A *balanced* diet of fresh, *natural* foods will improve kidney health as well as aid elimination. Plenty of water and fruit juices will dilute kidney wastes for easier elimination as well as have a cleansing, flushing effect.

How to Control the
Acid in Your Urine

Normally, the urine is slightly acid and contains a certain amount of solids (about five percent). Acid in the urine retards bacterial growth and helps to prevent infection. When the urine becomes overly acid, however, and contains an excessive amount of solids, trouble may develop. Concentrated urine can irritate the bladder, for example, or have a bad odor.

You can dilute and alkalize your urine simply by drinking plenty of water and fruit and vegetable juices. If you have an inflamed or infected bladder, or if urination causes burning pain, you should drink a glass of water or juice about every half hour. A little baking soda in water or lemonade will quickly alkalize your urine and help relieve pain during urination. You shouldn't use baking soda very often, however, since it neutralizes stomach acid and aggravates high blood pressure. Most fruits, such as apples, pears, peaches, lemons, oranges, grapes, figs, and raisins, will reduce the amount of acid in the urine. The acid in these fruits, after going through the body's metabolic process, leaves an alkaline ash that alkalizes the urine.

Note: Plums, prunes, cranberries, cereals, meats, eggs, fowl, and fish *increase* the amount of acid in the urine. You should go easy on these foods when your bladder or urinary tract is raw and inflamed.

**Special Care
for Kidney Trouble**

When the kidneys become diseased, treatment should be supervised by a doctor. Fortunately, it takes only about one-sixth of the total capacity of the kidneys to clear the blood of waste products. So there's a great deal of reserve for emergencies. It's very important, however, that special dietary recommendations be observed in the treatment of kidney troubles. The type of diet used will depend upon the type of trouble. In some cases, for example, protein intake will have to be restricted, while in others it may be necessary to increase the amount of protein in the diet. Obviously, you shouldn't attempt to treat kidney troubles yourself without the help of a physician.

Note: If your urine becomes smoky, cloudy, or discolored, or if your face and eyelids suddenly become swollen and puffy, see your doctor for a kidney examination.

If you urinate frequently and you feel weak, thirsty, and hungry, ask for a blood sugar test for diabetes.

Backache accompanied by fever is often the result of a kidney infection.

What to Do
About Kidney Stones

When kidney stones develop, it's essential to know what type of stones they are before adopting dietary measures.

Calcium phosphate stones, for example, call for a diet that's low in calcium and phosphorus. This means that it may be necessary to reduce your intake of milk fortified with Vitamin D. Alkalies or antacids should not be taken, especially with milk, since they may combine with calcium and contribute to the formation of stones.

Aluminum hydroxide gel, taken by mouth, unites with the phosphates in food to form aluminum phosphate, which is excreted by the bowels. The calcium eliminated by the urine will then be excreted in a form that will not harden to form stones.

Plenty of fluids will also reduce chances of stone formation by diluting the urine. Liberal use of meat, eggs, fowl, fish, and whole grain cereals and breads will help prevent the formation of calcium phosphate stones by increasing the acidity of the urine. Cranberries and plums are the only fresh fruits I know of that will increase the amount of acid in the urine.

Remember that inactivity results in loss of calcium from the bones. Excretion of this calcium through the kidneys can contribute to the formation of calcium phosphate stones. So be as active as possible — to keep your bones strong as well as to prevent kidney stones.

Calcium oxalate stones develop in an acid urine (below a pH of 7). Foods containing oxalic acid, such as rhubarb, spinach, cocoa, chocolate, wheat germ, and certain types of nuts, should be omitted from the diet. Liberal use of fruits and vegetables and their juices will *alkalize* the urine and reduce stone formation. Meats, fowl, eggs, fish, and cereals should be restricted. Milk intake should be limited to about one pint per day.

Oral supplements of magnesium and Vitamin B_6 (pyridoxine), along with about two quarts of water a day, have proven to be helpful in preventing the formation of oxalate stones.

Note: Because of the danger of calcium deficiency resulting from a "kidney stone diet," it's important to be examined periodically by a doctor.

FASTING: HOW TO LENGTHEN
YOUR LIFE BY RESTRICTING
YOUR DIET

Studies of longevity indicate that a low-calorie diet *lengthens* life, while a high-calorie diet *shortens* life. Also, there is some evidence to indicate that overfeeding a child to hasten growth and maturity will shorten his life. Anyone who has studied nutrition and the aging process has read of the experiments of the late Dr. Clive McCay of Cornell University, who doubled the life span of rats by underfeeding them. Rats that were fed adequate amounts of protein, vitamins, and minerals, but not enough calories to support normal growth, lived *twice as long* as rats that were fed an adequate diet that included sugar and lard.

Most of us overeat. Many of the excess calories we consume could be eliminated simply by avoiding refined and processed foods. Remember that you need the protein, vitamins, and minerals supplied by a balanced diet of natural foods. So while you might benefit from a short fast or from a reduction in the amount of food you eat, you should never go without eating for a long period of time. A prolonged fast, for example, could lead to nutritional deficiencies. Rapid loss of weight may result in a painful attack of gout. Insufficient carbohydrate for energy may cause illness (ketosis) from excessive burning of body fat. Stomach ulcers might develop from the action of stomach acid on an empty stomach. And so on.

Thus, while a *short fast* can be helpful in cleansing the body and the blood, a long fast can be harmful. Hunger pangs and a desire for food begin to disappear after three days of fasting. A person on a long fast can develop a serious nutritional deficiency and still not crave food. This is one of the biggest dangers of total fasting. Even with the use of supplements, a long fast can result in deficiencies.

A two-day fast will be long enough for most people. This will give the tissue cells enough time to dump accumulated wastes into the blood without developing a deficiency. You don't have to leave your stomach empty, however. Plenty of fruits, juices, and water during a fast from solid foods will aid the kidneys in eliminating wastes and help neutralize blood and urinary acids.

**How to Prepare
for a Two-Day Fast**

If you are accustomed to eating large amounts of food each day, it may not be a good idea to suddenly quit eating and go on a fast. It might be best to begin by tapering down the amount of food you eat. First eliminate *all* foods that are not nutritious natural foods. Ice cream, soft drinks, pastries, refined cereals, white bread, candy, spaghetti, and other refined or processed foods contribute calories without nutrients. Gradually reduce the amount of the other foods you eat. Eat the basic natural foods in progressively smaller but balanced amounts. After a couple of weeks, your stomach will have shrunk enough to prevent hunger pangs during a two-day fast. You may then leave off all solid foods except fruits. Plenty of water and juices will aid your kidneys in flushing out acid wastes.

After two days of fasting, you can begin eating small servings of the basic natural foods. You'll find that it won't take a large amount of food to fill your shrunken stomach. If you'll avoid overeating or stuffing yourself, so that you don't stretch your stomach to its former size, you can continue to eat smaller, low-calorie meals for a longer life. You may periodically repeat the two-day fast whenever you feel that you are getting toxic or sluggish. Regular use of basic food supplements will provide you with the nutritional insurance you need for good health.

Barton L. was constantly complaining about feeling sluggish and bloated. "I just don't feel good," he explained. "And I've always got a little headache." One look at his waistline and his eating habits suggested a toxic condition from overeating and a bad diet. I recommended a two-day fast from solid foods with liberal use of fruits, juices, and water. "I feel much better," Barton said at the end of the second day. "I have a lot more energy and I can think more clearly. In fact, all of my senses seem to be much sharper. I'm more alive and wide-awake than before."

Try the two-day fast yourself and see if it will revive your senses. Even if you don't feel bad, you can benefit from the cleansing and alkalizing effect of fruits and juices.

A LONG-RANGE
DIET FOR LONGEVITY

A short fast is a good cleanser, but for purposes of longevity you must adopt a long-range low-calorie diet made up of balanced amounts of the basic natural foods. Avoid refined and processed foods. If you like, you can supplement your diet with bone meal, Vitamins C and E, brewer's yeast, desiccated liver, fish liver oil, and other natural-food products. *The important thing is to reduce the number of calories in your diet without creating a deficiency in the essential food elements.* You must have adequate protein along with a certain amount of natural carbohydrates and a small amount of fat, supplied by *natural* foods that are rich in vitamins and minerals. Just be careful not to overeat.

SMOKING CAUSES
PREMATURE AGING AND DEATH

If you really want to be healthy and live a long time, you should not smoke tobacco. There is now considerable evidence to indicate that smoking causes premature aging as well as lung cancer and other fatal diseases.

Lung cancer. Every year, about 7,000 men die of lung cancer — and 90 percent of these are smokers. Women may be slightly more resistant to lung cancer because of the protective effect of certain hormones. With increasing numbers of women smoking, however, the incidence of lung cancer among women will increase. The tar in cigarette smoke contains about *30 different chemicals* that are capable of causing lung cancer.

Bronchitis and emphysema. According to the U.S. Public Health Service, there are over a million more cases of chronic bronchitis and emphysema than there would be if no one smoked. Emphysema is one of the fastest growing diseases in the United States. It is already killing about 30,000 Americans each year!

Heart attacks. The nicotine in cigarette smoke constricts the coronary arteries and speeds the heart rate. Whenever the effects of cigarette smoking are combined with exertion, emotional stress, hardened arteries, or heart disease, a reduction in the flow of blood to the heart muscle can result in sudden death from an apparent "heart attack."

Stomach ulcers. Swallowed smoke as well as the effects of nicotine absorbed into the blood can play a part in the development of ulcers in the stomach and small intestine. Even if you do not inhale cigarette smoke, nicotine absorbed through the mucous membranes of your mouth can affect the nerves that control the production of stomach acid.

Premature aging and wrinkling. Recent research has revealed that deep wrinkles in the face, particularly "crow's feet" at the corners of the eyes, can be caused by smoking cigarettes. The wrinkled face of a heavy smoker may make him look 20 years older than he really is.

Smoking may cause premature aging in many ways. It's well known that nicotine destroys Vitamin C in the blood. You need all the Vitamin C you can get to rebuild the collagen that holds your tissue cells together.

The tar from cigarette smoke coats the air sacs of the lungs and interferes with absorption of oxygen. The carbon monoxide in cigarette smoke also contributes to an oxygen deficiency by combining with red blood cells. Strangely enough, red blood cells will combine more readily with carbon monoxide than with oxygen. Simply breathing the smoke from someone else's cigarette can load your blood cells with carbon monoxide. So if you want to stay healthy and look young, stay out of smoke-filled rooms.

Sex and smoking. Some doctors have reported that persons who stop smoking experience renewed vigor and an increased desire for sex. If you aren't interested in giving up cigarettes just to be healthy so that you can live a long time, you might want to do so for a better sex life!

The longer you smoke, the greater your chances of dying young. It's never too late, however, to give up smoking. Many of the adverse effects of smoking can actually be reversed by quitting the habit. It's possible that ten years after you give up smoking, your health and life expectancy will be the same as that of a non-smoker.

HOW TO SWEAT OUT POISONS

Since the skin is an organ that eliminates waste from the body, you should make it a point to occasionally "work up a sweat." A few minutes of copious sweating will open the pores of the skin and flush out accumulated toxins. You can actually relieve the workload on your kidneys by sweating out nitrogen, urea, ammonia, and other waste products of protein metabolism. Harmful chemicals from foods and beverages and poisons from diseased organs are also eliminated by sweat.

Simple exercise affords the best way to stimulate perspiration. Exercise has the added benefit of strengthening your heart muscle. There are some special precautions to be observed, however, if you want to perspire safely and effectively.

You should never wear a plastic or rubber suit while exercising or perspiring. Sealing off your skin from circulating air may result in heat illness by causing a rise in body temperature. Remember that your body cannot cool itself if perspiration cannot evaporate freely from the skin. When the weather is hot, wear light, loose-fitting clothing, preferably a cotton fabric. Change the clothing when it becomes wet with sweat. About ten minutes of sweating will be enough to flush out your skin. Don't get too hot. Drink as much water as you want to satisfy your thirst. If you are active in sports and you perspire a lot, you may have to add one teaspoonful of salt to six quarts of drinking water in order to replace the salt you lose in your perspiration. Drink half a glass of the solution about every five minutes until your thirst is quenched.

Note: When the temperature is 90 to 100 degrees Fahrenheit with more than 70 percent relative humidity, or when the temperature is above 100 degrees, you should not make a deliberate effort to produce perspiration by exercising. When the temperature or the humidity is too high, your body may not be able to cool itself adequately. Dry air aids cooling by speeding the evaporation of sweat. But when the air is damp, sweat cannot evaporate and cooling is hindered. Obviously, you can stand a higher temperature when the air is dry than when the air is moist.

Don't be a weekend athlete! If you exercise to "work up a sweat," you should do so at least twice a week to condition your body against strain or injury.

FOOD ADDITIVES CAN
CLOG YOUR SYSTEM

Ordinarily, your liver can detoxify harmful substances that find their way into your system. With increasing use of artificial additives in foods, however, the accumulation of harmful chemicals in the body may soon become a major cause of premature aging, disease, and death. *About two or three thousand additives are now routinely added to food.* The average person consumes about five pounds of these additives each year!

The Surgeon General of the United States has testified that many commonly used food additives could have adverse effects on human health. The American Public Health Association has also warned that the increasing use of chemicals in food is a potential health hazard that might become one of the greatest problems the food industry has ever had to face.* So it's not just "food faddists" who are concerned about artificial additives in foods. It may be true that a few additives are helpful in

---

*The Chemical Feast, Grossman Publishers, New York, 1970.

maintaining the food supply in some parts of the country. Most food additives, however, are used to increase the profits of food manufacturers.

Once non-food chemicals get into your body, many of them cannot be eliminated. Instead, they may accumulate in joints, tissues, and organs to cause disease. Nothing is known about the long-range effects of many commonly-used additives. Although most additives have no obvious immediate effects, there are some that do result in unpleasant reactions. Monosodium glutamate and sodium nitrate, for example, have been known to cause headache.

Clifford B. suffered from recurring headache that did not respond to any form of treatment. Repeated medical examination failed to yield a diagnosis. I had just learned that certain food additives could cause headache, so I asked Clifford to keep a record of everything he ate for a week and to note the time when his headaches seemed to be worst. With a little detective work, we found that he developed a throbbing headache after eating meats preserved with nitrates and after eating at a steak house where the meat was heavily seasoned with monosodium glutamate. When he avoided foods containing these additives, his headaches disappeared!

The only way you can avoid artificial food additives is to eat fresh, natural foods. Steer clear of processed or synthetic foods whenever possible. No matter how "enriched" a processed food may be, don't buy it if it contains artificial additives. Avoid meats and other foods that contain preservatives. Most grocery stores now sell bread, cereals, and other basic foods that are completely natural. Any supermarket can supply you with the fresh fruits, vegetables, meats, eggs, milk, juices, cheeses, nuts, grains, dried foods, and other products you need for a wholesome, balanced diet. *Careful selection of the foods you eat will reward you with better health and prolong your life.*

HOW TO IMPROVE THE
FUNCTION OF YOUR LIVER

In addition to filtering toxins and wastes from your blood, your liver manufactures blood, supplies fuel, assembles food elements for rebuilding tissue, stores vitamins and minerals, and produces important enzymes. When the liver is not functioning properly, toxins accumulate in the blood to cause fatigue and premature aging. Hemorrhoids, varicose veins, and swollen ankles may develop from obstruction of blood flow through the liver. Remember that *all* of the blood circulating through the body must pass through the liver for cleansing and servicing.

Note: The appearance of large, prominent veins on the abdomen, radiating from the naval, may mean that there is serious circulatory obstruction in the liver. Jaundice, in which the skin and the eyeballs turn yellow, may mean that the liver is diseased. Be sure to bring these symptoms to the attention of your doctor.

Improve Circulation with a Liver Pack

You can stimulate the function of your liver by using a special pack to increase the flow of blood through your liver.

Put a little mustard or oil of wintergreen into a pan of hot water. Fold a large, thick towel several times, soak it in the water, and then wring it out just enough to prevent dripping. Place the towel over your liver (just beneath the ribs on the right side of your abdomen) and cover it with a sheet of rubber or plastic to hold in the heat and moisture. A hot water bottle placed over the pack will keep it hot.

After about 20 minutes, remove the pack and sponge the skin with cold water.

The circulatory reaction of the water treatment, and the effect of mustard or wintergreen on the skin, will have a long-lasting effect on the circulation of blood through the liver. Just be careful not to use so much mustard or wintergreen that you blister your skin.

Summary

1. The elimination of waste by the bowels, lungs, skin, and kidneys prevents accumulation of toxins that cause fatigue, premature aging, disease, and death.
2. Visiting the toilet regularly, eating foods that are

rich in cellulose, and drinking plenty of liquids will relieve constipation and prevent the accumulation of waste in the colon.

3. When the bowels fail to empty after three or four days, a simple enema will help restore regularity.

4. When the bladder and urethra are raw and inflamed, you should reduce the acidity of your urine by drinking fruit and vegetable juices.

5. An acid urine helps prevent the formation of calcium phosphate stones, while an alkaline urine helps prevent formation of calcium oxalate stones.

6. A two-day fast from solid foods, with liberal use of fruits, juices, and water, will have a cleansing effect on the body.

7. A *low-calorie diet* that provides adequate amounts of vitamins, minerals, protein, carbohydrate, and fat is an important key to longevity.

8. Smoking cigarettes causes premature aging as well as such diseases as lung cancer, emphysema, and stomach ulcers.

9. "Working up a sweat" flushes toxins out of the skin and relieves the workload on the kidneys.

10. Refined and processed foods often contain artificial additives that harm the liver and accumulate in the body to cause premature aging and disease.

LIFE EXTENDER #8

How to Restore Youthful
Digestion Virtually Overnight

No matter how careful you are about selecting the foods you eat, you won't get all the nutrients you need for a long, healthy life if your digestion is faulty. Everything you eat must be broken down by digestive juices so that the essential nutrients can be absorbed. Once the nutrients reach the circulating blood, they are transported throughout the body and used to build and repair living cells. Some of the nutrients are reassembled in the liver to form a variety of substances needed by the body.

Once you are sure that your diet contains all the essential nutrients, there is much that you can do to assure their absorption.

DIGESTION BEGINS WITH CHEWING

You don't have to chew every bite of food a certain number of times, as once advocated by some food faddists. There are, however, several good reasons why you should chew your food thoroughly. Saliva, for example, contains an alkaline enzyme that aids in the digestion of starches and carbohydrates. The effectiveness of this enzyme depends upon how well you chew your food. Also, if every morsel of food you eat is crushed by your teeth, the digestive enzymes in the stomach and the small intestine can act effectively in preparing protein, carbohydrate, and fat for absorption.

Swallowing large hunks of food prevents normal digestion and may contribute to such digestive disturbances as gas, cramps, or diarrhea. People who bolt their food down hurriedly may develop nutritional deficiencies as well as suffer from digestive disturbances. So it's very important that you chew your food thoroughly. Make sure that you allow yourself enough time to eat your meals *slowly*. If a dental problem makes it difficult or impossible to chew your food properly, see your dentist as soon as possible. It takes a full set of teeth, natural or artificial, to chew the fruits, vegetables, and meats you need for healthy longevity.

HOW TO HELP YOUR STOMACH

When food reaches the stomach, hydrochloric acid and other juices begin the digestion of protein. (If food has been adequately chewed, the alkaline enzymes in the saliva do their job *before* the food reaches the acid environment of the stomach.) There are several things that you can do to aid your stomach in completing its work.

First of all, try to be tranquil and relaxed when you eat your meals. Any kind of emotional excitement can inhibit the function of your stomach. Nicotine from cigarette smoke may also delay emptying of your stomach. So don't smoke just before eating.

Don't overeat. Overloading your stomach may force it to empty prematurely, making it difficult or impossible for the small intestine to complete the digestive process. Enzymes released into the small intestine by the pancreas aid in the digestion of protein, carbohydrate, and fat, but the small intestine is alkaline and cannot adequately break down strands of meat. Intestinal absorption of undigested protein may result in an allergic reaction, causing hives, a rash, or some other disorder.

Remember: *Be calm, eat slowly, chew your food thoroughly, and don't overeat.* Food properly chewed and digested will enable you to get more benefit from less food by supplying *more nutrients with fewer calories.* It's better to eat three or four small meals than to eat one or two large meals.

Foods should always be prepared and served in an appetizing manner. When food smells good, looks good, and tastes good, the flow of gastric juices is greatly stimulated, aiding digestion and absorption of nutrients. Macbeth's observation that "good digestion waits on appetite and health on both" is a truth for all to heed.

How to Aid Digestion with Supplements

If you continue to have digestive troubles in spite of careful attention to your eating habits, you may be deficient in digestive enzymes. Fortunately, there are some special supplements that you can use, and some special steps that you can take, to assure adequate digestion of food.

Stay Away from Alkalizers!

Many people assume that all you need for "indigestion" is an alkalizer to neutralize stomach acid. Actually, indigestion is caused more often by a *deficiency* in stomach acid than by an excess. And the older you become the more likely you are to be deficient in stomach acid. When "indigestion" occurs after eating, it's very likely that you need *more* stomach acid to digest the food in your stomach. Persons who take an alkalizer for indigestion caused by overeating may increase their discomfort by neutralizing the hydrochloric acid manufactured by the stomach.

Don't be too hasty about taking antacids and alkalizers for indigestion caused by eating. In addition to interfering with digestion, unnecessary use of alkalizers will neutralize the stomach acid you need to absorb calcium, iron, and other minerals. If you're over forty years of age, there's a good chance that your indigestion can be relieved by taking a hydrochloric acid supplement with your meals.

One of my patients, 60 year old Douglas G., suffered from such severe indigestion that he was occasionally unable to attend a business meeting because of painful cramps and spasms. Everytime he ate a meal, he took a popular, much-advertised alkalizer in anticipation of the belching, sour stomach, and gas pains that he knew would follow. Although the alkalizer never seemed to help, Douglas had been convinced by television advertising that he could not eat without taking something to "help his stomach." When I finally persuaded him to quit taking his customary after-dinner alkalizer, his cramps and spasms disappeared. When he supplemented his meals with hydrochloric acid tablets, *all* of his digestive problems disappeared!

How to Take
Hydrochloric Acid Supplements

Hydrochloric acid as a digestive aid may be taken in tablet or liquid form. You can purchase glutamic or betaine hydrochloric acid tablets in health food stores. Or you can get diluted (0.1 N) hydrochloric from a drug store. The tablets may simply be swallowed with meals. The acid in diluted liquid form must be diluted even more by mixing one teaspoonful in half a glass of water. The mixture may then be sipped through a glass straw. Be sure to place the straw well inside your mouth, on top of your tongue, so that the acid won't damage your teeth. Sip the mixture slowly with meals.

If your digestion seems to improve after taking hydrochloric acid with your meals, you may continue the practice. If your symptoms are aggravated, however, you may not need the additional acid.

Sipping apple cider or lemon juice solutions with meals will often aid digestion. Pineapple and papaya contain enzymes that aid in the digestion of protein. Many commercial meat tenderizers contain extract from the papaya plant.

When to Take
Pancreatic Enzymes

When symptoms of indigestion are accompanied by intestinal gas and clay-colored stools, there may be a deficiency in bile or pancreatic enzymes. Undigested fat in the stool, which gives it the clay color, may also mean that some of the fat-soluble vitamins are being lost. Supplements containing lecithin, ox bile, and pancreatic enzymes might help this situation. You should first check with your doctor, however, to rule out disease of the liver, the gall bladder, or the pancreas.

Note: Your health food store can supply you with a supplement containing hydrochloric acid, bile, and pancreatic enzymes — all in one tablet.

HOW TO OVERCOME
MILK ALLERGY WITH
FERMENTED MILK PRODUCTS

Lydia B. complained about gas pains and chronic diarrhea. "I teach high school English," she said, "and it's embarrassing to have to leave my class so frequently to go to the bathroom." Repeated examination by a number of doctors had failed to yield a diagnosis, and treatment had been unsuccessful. When she eliminated milk from her diet, her bowel problems disappeared virtually overnight. "Since I quit having milk with my breakfast cereal," she reported, "I haven't had to leave my class a single time."

Milk is a common cause of digestive or bowel disturbances in adults. It seems that many adults do not have the digestive enzymes (lactase) they need to digest milk sugar (lactose). As a result, the milk they drink causes intestinal gas or diarrhea. When milk has been fermented, however, to make yogurt, buttermilk, or cottage cheese, the lactose is converted to lactic acid. If you suspect that milk is giving you trouble, switch to *fermented* milk products.

Remember that any type of diarrhea, whether caused by milk allergy or disease, results in loss of essential nutrients.

HOW TO COPE
WITH ACUTE DIARRHEA

When diarrhea begins, try drinking cultured buttermilk or eating bananas. Buttermilk is rich in friendly bacteria and lactic acid, which may help restore the normal environment of the colon. Bananas contain pectin, which absorbs and eliminates poisons. Many popular remedies for diarrhea, such as Kaopectate and Pectocil, contain fruit pectin, which soaks up poisons in the intestinal tract.

When diarrhea is so severe that everything you eat and drink is quickly eliminated, it may be necessary to fast 12 to 24 hours in order to relieve the load on your intestines. As soon as possible, however, you should begin taking salty soups and broths to replace the salt and water lost through your bowels. Without an adequate intake of fluids, prolonged diarrhea can result in dangerous dehydration. So the sooner you can take fluids the better.

Water-retention enema. Persons who are suffering from both vomiting and diarrhea may be able to benefit from a water-retention enema. Several ounces of water are injected into the rectum and held as long as possible. Some of the water will be absorbed by the body. When the remaining water is expelled, it will washout toxins that may be irritating the colon. In any event, enough water will be absorbed to prevent serious dehydration.

HOW TO CONTROL DIVERTICULITIS

It's now believed that excessive use of refined carbohydrates clogs and stretches the bowel until tiny ballooned-out pouches or diverticula form on the wall of the colon. When these pouches become clogged and inflamed, painful abdominal cramps with constipation or diarrhea may occur. More than a third of Americans over the age of forty have pouches on their colon. With more and more Americans eating refined and processed foods, it's safe to assume that the incidence of diverticulitis will increase as the years go by.

If you don't already have pouches on your colon, you may be able to *prevent* their development by eating foods containing cellulose. All types of fruits and vegetables contain cellulose or indigestible fibers that will sweep your colon clean. When there is adequate cellulose in your intestinal tract, the fibers will retain moisture and prevent packing of waste matter. This will prevent constipation and allow easy and efficient evacuation of your bowels.

Eat something raw every day. When you cook vegetables,

put some aside for use in raw salads. Keep a variety of fresh fruits in your home so that you can have a fruit snack each evening before retiring.

A Temporary Diet
for Diverticulitis

When the bowel becomes inflamed by an acute attack of diverticulitis, it may be necessary to temporarily discontinue the use of raw and coarse foods until the symptoms subside. Fruits and vegetables may have to be cooked or pureed to soften them a little. Milk, eggs, cheese, meat, and other soft foods can be eaten safely.

The juices of raw fruits and vegetables can supply important vitamins and enzymes. If you puree fruits and vegetables, be sure to strain out all seeds and husks.

If your diet must be severely restricted, it might be a good idea to include a little agar or psyllium seed extract for mois-ture-retaining bulk. It's very important to avoid constipation, since pressure in the bowels will increase the size of the pouches.

When symptoms subside and you are once again able to eat fresh fruits and salads, you should continue to avoid bran, seeds, husks, and other indigestible particles that might accumulate in intestinal pouches. Remember, however, that you need a certain amount of cellulose to retain moisture and clean your bowels. Cellulose also encourages the growth of friendly bacteria.

HOW TO SPEED
HEALING OF STOMACH ULCERS

No one knows for sure what causes a stomach ulcer. We do know, however, that an ulcer does not occur in the absence of acid. When there is an excessive amount of stomach acid, or a deficiency in the mucus that protects the lining of the stomach, raw spots develop that allow the development of an ulcer. A gnawing, burning pain that develops when the stomach is empty usually means that stomach acid is reaching a raw spot. If bleeding occurs, the stool will be black. Any evidence of bleeding should be brought to the attention of a physician.

There are certain foods that must be avoided during the acute stages of an ulcer, but most doctors now feel that there is no specific diet that heals stomach ulcers. Some doctors allow ulcer patients to eat whatever they feel agrees with them. There is now some evidence to indicate that with sensible eating habits and freedom from emotional stress an ulcer will heal itself. In any event, *most ulcers will heal if they can be spared contact with undiluted stomach acid for several weeks.* This means frequent feeding of special foods to absorb the acid secreted by the stomach. High-protein meals with a snack every two hours is usually best. Protein foods such as broiled meat, fish, poultry, eggs, milk, yogurt, or cottage cheese will absorb stomach acid more readily than starchy foods.

You should avoid plain soup and meat broths, since they stimulate the production of stomach acid without neutralizing the acid. Cream soups, however, containing milk and pureed vegetables, might be helpful in the treatment of a painful ulcer.

Coffee, tea, alcohol, tobacco, raw vegetables, fried or spicy foods, and coarse breads and cereals that might irritate or scratch a raw, painful ulcer should be avoided. Hourly feedings of milk and crackers, creamy cereals, cornstarch puddings, or soft-boiled eggs may be necessary to relieve pain. If constipation occurs while a soft diet is being used to avoid aggravating a painful ulcer, milk of magnesia may have beneficial laxative and antacid effects.

If you use food to neutralize stomach acid, you won't need to take commercial antacids. If you do take antacids, be sure not to take them with milk. Combining milk and alkali will interfere with the absorption and use of calcium and may even result in the formation of kidney stones.

How to Use Milk
to Ease Ulcer Pain

Milk is often used to relieve the pain of a stomach ulcer. The protein in milk absorbs stomach acid, while the fat in milk protects the lining of the stomach from the corrosive effects of the acid. Too much milk fat, however, may increase the amount of hard fat and cholesterol in the blood as well as contribute to a build-up of body fat. Skim milk may be adequate for relieving the pain of a stomach ulcer, but the milk will stay in the stomach longer if it contains fat. Rather than drink whole milk, which is rich in saturated fat, you might want to add a little vegetable oil to skim milk.

How to Make
Vegetable Oil Milk

Mix 1½ tablespoons of honey and one teaspoonful of powdered egg white into 12 ounces of skim milk in a blender. While mixing at a slow speed, pour in six tablespoons of corn oil. Then add 12 more ounces of skim milk. A banana may be added for flavor. A little powdered skim milk may be added for extra protein. (Remember that stomach acid acts primarily on protein. The oil coats the stomach and delays digestion while the protein absorbs the acid.)

How to Make Soy Milk

If you are allergic to the lactose in milk, you can drink buttermilk or soy milk. To make soy milk, blend one cup of full-fat soy flour and one third cup of calcium lactate with one quart of water. Honey may be added for flavor, and one egg white may be added for its antacid effect.

How to Make
a Home Alkalizer

When you are suffering from the pain of a stomach ulcer and there is no food available to absorb the acid, you can make an effective alkalizer. All you have to do is dip up just enough sodium bicarbonate to cover the tip of a spoon and then stir it into a glass of water. Sip the mixture slowly. Too large a dose taken too rapidly will only cause an acid rebound, in which the stomach produces more acid to overcome the alkalizing effect of the soda. (A banana or a little creamy cereal containing a teaspoonful of fruit pectin, eaten one-half hour after taking soda, will absorb any acid rebound.)

Don't get into the habit of taking soda every day. Sodium bicarbonate can be absorbed into your system, resulting in illness caused by alkalosis. Commercial antacids are not ab-

sorbed by the body, but they may cause constipation or diarrhea. So whenever possible, it's best to use *food* to absorb
stomach acid rather than try to neutralize it with an antacid.
Remember that excessive or unnecessary use of alkalizers will
interfere with the absorption of vitamins and minerals by the
stomach.

Note: While stomach ulcers can occur at any age, they occur
most often before the arrival of middle age. So the older you
become the less likely you are to develop an ulcer. In fact, it's
more likely that you will develop a deficiency in stomach acid.

Alcohol, Coffee, Cigarettes, and Drugs
Can Aggravate Stomach Ulcers

Alcohol. A small amount of alcohol, such as an occasional
glass of wine with dinner, may aid digestion by stimulating the
appetite and relieving nervous tension. Excessive use of alcohol, however, especially on an empty stomach, can inflame the
stomach and lead to the development of gastritis. It can also
aggravate stomach ulcers by increasing the production of stomach acid. Prolonged use of alcohol destroys the B vitamins you
need for a healthy nervous system.

So while an occasional cocktail with dinner may be harmless
or even beneficial, you should not drink very often or between
meals. If you have a stomach ulcer, you should not drink at all!

Coffee. The caffeine in coffee can aggravate stomach ulcers
by causing the stomach to produce an excessive amount of acid.
Caffeine is absorbed into the blood where it reaches the nerve
centers that control the production of acid. For this reason, I
usually advise ulcer patients not to drink coffee.

If you must drink coffee, drink it *after* eating, or drink
decaffeinated coffee.

Note: Tea and cola drinks also contain caffeine.

Cigarettes. Cigarette smoking has been directly connected
with the development of stomach ulcers. Since nothing good
can be said about smoking, you should not smoke at all —
even if you do not have an ulcer. The nicotine from cigarette
smoke can actually interfere with digestion by slowing down
the muscular action of the stomach and the intestines. Swallow-

ing smoke can have a harmful effect on the lining of the stomach.

Drugs. The use of cortisone in the treatment of arthritis can greatly aggravate stomach ulcers by producing an overflow of stomach acid. If you are undergoing treatment for arthritis, be sure to tell your doctor if you have an ulcer. The salicylic acid of aspirin can also aggravate an ulcer by inflaming the lining of the stomach. Be careful about taking any kind of drug.

How to Relieve Stomach Ulcers with Rest, Sleep, and Sex

Rest and sleep. Plenty of rest and sleep are essential in the treatment of a stomach ulcer. When the body is relaxed and the mind is tranquil, the stomach produces less acid. It may be necessary, however, to have a bedtime snack followed by another snack or two during the night to keep stomach acid neutralized.

Sex. Regular sexual intercourse can be a great tension reliever when it involves a compatible, loving couple. When performed with a complaining, resentful mate, however, it can cause a great deal of emotional stress and anxiety. Few activities have such potential for both good and bad as sex in marriage. If you suffer from nervous tension or have a stomach ulcer, and you have a thoughtful, loving, and active mate, you should take full advantage of the medicinal value of sex.

Did you know that a pregnant woman never develops a stomach ulcer? And that pregnancy heals a woman's ulcers? The reason for this is not known, but it probably has something to do with the production of hormones.

HOW TO CULTIVATE HELPFUL BACTERIA IN YOUR COLON

Ordinarily, the intestinal tract contains large amounts of friendly bacteria that aid the digestive process and prevent the growth of hostile or disease-producing bacteria. When these bacteria are destroyed by oral antibiotics or by excessive use of laxatives, digestion and elimination are hindered and colon problems develop. If you suffer from constipation, gas, putrefaction, colitis, and other problems of the lower bowel, you may be suffering from a bacterial deficiency in your colon.

Yogurt made from lactobacillus acidophilus is loaded with friendly bacteria that can destroy the unfriendly bacteria in your colon by producing lactic acid. Once the acidophilus bacteria have been planted in your intestine, they will continue to multiply if your diet contains lactose or milk sugar. (Whey is rich in milk sugar.) If you are allergic to milk sugar, and the use of milk causes gas or diarrhea, you should continue to eat cultured yogurt occasionally in order to keep your colon supplied with bacteria. Remember that yogurt is rich in lactic acid and low in lactose.

You can purchase pure yogurt in health food stores or you can make your own. Simply adding a little yogurt to fresh milk will produce a new batch of yogurt in 24 hours or so. Or you can add acidophilus culture to milk to make yogurt from scratch. (See Life Extender #1 for instructions on how to make yogurt.)

HINTS FOR GALL
BLADDER SUFFERERS

When we think of digestion, we think primarily of the stomach. Much "indigestion," however, may result from a "bad gall bladder." Actually, the gall bladder is simply a reservoir for bile, which is manufactured by the liver. When fat leaves the stomach and enters the small intestine, the gall bladder empties its contents into the intestine, mixing bile with fat. Lecithin in the bile breaks the fat into tiny particles so that the fat can be absorbed.

When there is not sufficient bile flow, the fat passes through the intestinal tract unabsorbed (causing clay-colored stools), taking calcium, iron, and fat-soluble Vitamins A, D, E, and K along with it. (Calcium and iron combine with undigested fat to form hard soap.) This can lead to anemia, constipation, brittle bones, collapsed vertebrae, night blindness, and other diseases, not to mention digestive disturbances. A coating of

unabsorbed fat in the small intestine may also prevent digestion of protein and carbohydrate.

How to Empty the Gall Bladder

Most people with "gall bladder trouble" try to avoid fatty
foods, for fear of having "bilious indigestion." Actually, there
should be a certain amount of fat in the diet to stimulate emptying of the gall bladder, otherwise the fat-soluble vitamins
won't be absorbed. So while you should avoid fried foods,
greasy soups, and animal fat, you need a little of the right kind
of fat. (If your gall bladder does not empty each day, gall stones
may form.)

A small amount of vegetable oil with meals will stimulate a
sluggish gall bladder and supply the essential fatty acids your
liver needs to produce lecithin for bile. A tablespoonful of
corn oil, olive oil, or safflower oil, for example, can be put on
toast, in a green salad, or in a glass of warm milk. Lecithin and
bile tablets may be taken with fatty meals.

How to Avoid Surgery
for Gall Stones

It has been estimated that 16 million Americans have gall
stones. Not all gall stones cause trouble, however, and most
people are not aware that they have them. When a stone blocks
the gall bladder, causing pain, spasm, bloating, belching, and
complete intolerance to fatty foods, surgery may be needed to
relieve the symptoms. You should always seek the opinion of
at least two specialists in internal medicine before submitting
to surgery. It's unfortunately true that many "physicians and
surgeons" will remove a gall bladder unnecessarily. It's not
necessary to remove a gall bladder simply because it contains
stones. Of course, when a stone becomes impacted in the neck
or duct of a gall bladder, the pain and other symptoms will be
so severe and so persistent as to leave little doubt about the
need for surgery.

Note: Blocking of a bile passage by a stone occurs most

often at about 50 or 60 years of age, and more commonly in women than in men.

How to Recognize the
Symptoms of a Gall Stone

When a stone becomes lodged in the duct of the gall bladder, severe pain just under the ribs on the right side of the abdomen may radiate into the right shoulder or into the back just beneath the right shoulder blade. There may also be fever, chills, nausea, abdominal distension, and jaundice, with extreme tenderness over the area of the gall bladder. Since the pain may last for several hours, it's best to see a doctor as soon as possible for appropriate medication.

How to Prevent
and Dissolve Gall Stones

No one knows for sure what causes gall stones, but since most of the stones are made up of cholesterol, dietary measures might be helpful in dissolving the stones or preventing their formation. A high-protein diet that's low in animal fat and balanced with fruits and vegetables will help prevent a build-up of blood fat and body fat. Supplements containing lecithin, B vitamins, and Vitamin E will help keep cholesterol stones from forming. A little vegetable oil daily will supply essential fatty acids (which combat a build-up of cholesterol) as well as force the gall bladder to empty. Hydrogenated vegetable fat, fried and greasy foods, and processed foods should be completely avoided.

Eat three meals a day. Nibbling all day to satisfy your appetite may not stimulate your gall bladder enough to empty its stored bile. Remember that an inactive gall bladder tends to concentrate its contents and form stones. Drink plenty of water each day so that you'll have adequate fluid for the formation of bile.

HOW TO HANDLE
AN IRRITABLE COLON

Clyde B. was a busy attorney who had a great deal of responsibility in handling the legal affairs of several industrial firms.

"My bowels are driving me crazy," he complained. "I'm always having stomach cramps and gas pains. And when I'm not constipated, I have diarrhea. My doctors can't find anything wrong with me."

Clyde was suffering from an irritable colon. Nervous tension, worry, hurried meals, overwork, and inadequate sleep had disturbed the function of his colon by upsetting his nervous system. His colon had simply gone "haywire," sometimes speeding up and sometimes slowing down. As a result, he suffered from constipation followed by diarrhea that drained partially-digested food from his intestinal tract. All of this resulted in abdominal rumbling and painful spasms. Nausea, loss of appetite, belching, and heartburn were setting the stage for the development of a stomach ulcer. "And, that's not all," Clyde added. "Sometimes I feel weak and light-headed. I have headaches, my heart pounds, I can't sleep at night, and I occasionally break out in a heavy sweat."

And no wonder. Clyde's bowel was depriving him of nutrients and upsetting his entire system. *All of this was the result of a nervous storm created by emotional and physical stress.*

Any type of unrelieved emotional stress or anxiety can disturb the digestive system. It's very important that you avoid the type of work schedule that keeps you worried and aggravated 24 hours a day. Always allow enough time in each day for rest and recreation. Control your working hours so that you don't overwork. And when the day's work is done, forget it. Physical exercise is often very effective in relieving tension, relaxing muscles, and getting your mind off your problems.

Clyde was so deeply rooted in his daily "rat race" that he found it impossible to relax enough to slowdown and sleep. I advised him to drop one or two of his clients, take a week off, and then start over with controlled, abbreviated working hours. He was instructed to set aside enough time each day for recreation and total relaxation. After a few weeks on such a schedule, with a daily diet of fresh, natural foods, Clyde's problems disappeared. "I feel like a new man," he said with an obvious new grip on life. "I never realized that the mind could have such an effect on the bowels."

You should try to follow Clyde's example. You can prevent the emotional and nervous storm that wrecks your stomach and your bowels. Remember that if digestion and elimination are so faulty that your body is deprived of essential nutrients, you'll suffer from disease and die prematurely.

Watch Out for Colitis and Sprue

When diarrhea is persistent or accompanied by bloody or frothy stools, see your doctor for a checkup. Ulcerative colitis, colon tumors, and other serious conditions require close medical supervision.

Allergy to milk, wheat, and eggs has been known to cause ulcerative colitis.

Persons who are deficient in the enzyme they need to digest gluten, a protein substance found in wheat, rye, oats, and barley, suffer a fatty diarrhea (non-tropical sprue) that drains the body of fat-soluble vitamins and minerals. Treatment requires a special diet that excludes all foods and beverages made with grains that contain gluten. Only flour products made from rice, corn, potatoes, and soybeans can be used.

Summary

1. Adequate chewing of food assures digestion of carbohydrates and prepares protein and fats for the action of stomach and intestinal secretions.
2. Persons deficient in stomach acid and digestive juices can improve digestion by taking a supplement containing hydrochloric acid, ox bile, and pancreatic enzymes.
3. Persistent diarrhea accompanied by clay-colored stools should be brought to the attention of a specialist in internal medicine.
4. Diets that are rich in refined carbohydrates and deficient in cellulose supplied by fruits and vegetables can lead to diverticulitis by packing and stretching the colon.
5. Most stomach ulcers will heal in several weeks if

protein-rich foods and beverages are used often enough to absorb excess stomach acid.

6. Caffeine in coffee and nicotine in cigarettes can lead to indigestion and stomach ulcers through their effect on the central nervous system.

7. Yogurt and fermented milk products made with lactobacillus acidophilus aid digestion and improve elimination by supplying friendly bacteria for the intestinal tract.

8. Persons with a sluggish gall bladder should avoid meat fat and fried and greasy foods and use vegetable oil to stimulate the flow of bile.

9. Supplements containing lecithin, Vitamin E, Vitamin B complex, and the essential fatty acids (vegetable oil) produce bile and prevent the formation of gall stones.

10. Overwork, emotional stress, hurried meals, and inadequate sleep can lead to indigestion as well as to disturbed colon function.

LIFE EXTENDER #9

The New, Natural Way
to Reduce Body Fat and
Improve Your Physical Appearance

Overweight, poor posture, and inactivity are common causes of disease and premature aging. Simple steps taken to remove these aging influences will improve your physical appearance as well as lengthen your life. With Life Extender #9, you'll learn how to *eat* to reduce excess body fat, and how to improve your health by improving your body mechanics. Even if you aren't overweight, the "reducing diet" I recommend can be used to assure continued good health and an ideal bodyweight.

STAY SLIM AND
TRIM AND LIVE LONGER

Remember when mothers used to brag about who had the fattest baby? People once believed that a fat baby was always a healthy baby. We now know that an excessive amount of body fat contributes to the development of disease — *and a fat baby usually becomes a fat adult.* Once extra fat cells form in the body of a child, they remain for a lifetime, always ready to gobble up excess calories in the diet. So if you were one of mom's prize fat babies, you'll have more trouble than the average person in controlling your bodyweight. It's very important, however, that you take whatever measures necessary to rid your body of excess fat. There's no longer any doubt that obesity contributes to the development of disease and premature aging. Life insurance studies, for example, indicate that overweight persons are more apt to suffer from high blood pressure, cardiovascular disease, cancer, diabetes, kidney ailments, arthritis, hernia, gall bladder trouble, and other common ailments.

In addition to causing such diseases as atherosclerosis, there is some evidence to indicate that an excessive amount of animal fat in the diet shortens life expectancy in some other unknown way. A group of nutritionists who made a long-term study of 97 middle-aged and elderly women found that those who had the highest intake of fat had the shortest life span. "It is conceivable," they concluded, "that food fats inadvertently may carry some noxious agent."*

So even if you are slim and apparently healthy, it might be a good idea to cut down on all types of fat in your diet. Hardened arteries caused by animal fat may occur without any apparent increase in body fat. No matter how much you weigh, you must limit your intake of fat. If you have an excessive amount of body fat, you must limit your intake of both carbohydrate and fat. Most people who are too fat eat excessive amounts of refined carbohydrates.

The natural food diet recommended in this chapter will automatically balance the protein, carbohydrate, and fat in your diet. You can literally eat your way to a new and youthful body and still enjoy all the pleasures of eating. It's simply a matter of eating *properly.*

Note: You don't need to consult a height-weight chart to determine whether or not you are too fat. A view of your

---

*"Nutrition and Health of Older People," by Schlenker, et al., *The American Journal of Clinical Nutrition,* October, 1973.

nude body in a mirror will give you the answer. If you can pinch up more than an inch of fat on the back of your upper arm, you need to reduce your bodyweight. Nearly 40 percent of all Americans are overweight!

WHY NATURAL FOODS ARE
SUPERIOR TO REFINED FOODS

There is now some evidence to indicate that natural foods are not as fattening as refined foods. One reason for this is that natural foods are digested and absorbed more slowly than refined foods, and they contain the elements your body needs to utilize the nutrients they supply. Refined foods, on the other hand, are so highly concentrated in carbohydrate and empty calories that they are quickly absorbed into the blood stream. This results in a flood of blood sugar that forces the body to store much of the sugar as fat, leaving very little to be burned as energy. This is why persons who eat excessive amounts of refined foods are usually tired, hungry, unhealthy, and *fat*.

If you are to be successful in controlling your bodyweight, you must avoid refined foods, especially those containing sugar or white flour. In addition to packing fat on your body, refined carbohydrates contribute to the development of arthritis, hardened arteries, and colon cancer. Simply eliminating refined foods from your diet may be all that you need to do to reduce your bodyweight. Remember that even if you are not fat, you should not eat refined carbohydrates if you want to be healthy and free from disease. On a diet of natural foods, you can actually eat more without gaining weight, and you'll be less likely to overeat. Natural foods do not artificially stimulate the appetite, and they do not overpower the appetite mechanism that controls your intake of calories.

How Rachel G. Solved Her
Overweight Problem with Natural Foods

"I eat less than most people," Rachel G. claimed, "but I still gain weight." An analysis of Rachel's diet revealed that she ate predominately starchy foods, such as pancakes, sandwiches, spaghetti, pizza, potatoes, and so on. Her meals prepared at home consisted of canned, packaged, and frozen

"TV dinners" that were loaded with empty calories. She had frequent snacks of cookies and other sweets. Rachel never purchased fresh fruits and vegetables. She didn't believe in taking vitamins. "I wouldn't be caught dead in a health food store," she announced.

Actually, Rachel was already nearly dead. In addition to being obese, she suffered from arthritis. Her hair was thin and brittle, her complexion pasty. Constipation, kidney infections, skin problems, and a host of other complaints forced her to make frequent trips to doctors' offices. Rachel looked bad and felt bad. She was a terror in public and an apparition in bed. She was clearly nutritionally deficient. It was true that she didn't eat as much as most people, but what she did eat was rich in calories and low in nutrients.

All of Rachel's problems were the result of bad eating habits. When I finally convinced her that she could reduce her bodyweight and improve her health simply by eating fresh, natural foods, she agreed to follow my instructions. In just a few months, she began to look better and feel better. The fat gradually melted from her body, and she made fewer trips to doctors' offices. After about a year, she was a healthy-looking woman. A "natural foods reducing diet" can do as much for you.

How to Select Natural
Foods on a Reducing Diet

A natural foods reducing diet is really very simple to follow. All you have to do is eat low-fat natural foods. To begin with, this means eating *lean meats* that have been trimmed of all visible fat before baking, broiling, or roasting. *Chicken* and most varieties of *fish* are low in saturated fat. The skin of a chicken, however, is rich in fat and should be discarded *before* cooking. Chicken, fish, or lean meat may be eaten generously at each meal. You need plenty of protein on any kind of reducing diet. *Skim milk* and *uncreamed cottage cheese* are good sources of low-fat protein.

In order to make sure that you get the carbohydrate, vitamins, and minerals you need, you should eat a *fresh, green salad* and two *fresh vegetables* each day. Make sure that the vegetables are cooked without grease or oil. You can get the essential fatty acids you need by mixing a little vegetable oil with vinegar for use as a salad dressing.

A beverage with each meal, preferably *water, skim milk or vegetable juice,* won't interfere with digestion and will help satisfy your appetite. Finish your meal with *fresh or dried fruit* for dessert.

Breakfast will give you an opportunity to eat *whole grain cereals* along with fruit, lean ham or Canadian bacon, juice, and other low-fat, natural foods.

In the course of a day, you should eat some of *all* the basic natural foods to assure an adequate intake of essential nutrients. If every meal is made up of natural foods, chances are you'll be able to satisfy your appetite without overeating. Overweight persons who are accustomed to eating measured amounts of processed foods are often surprised to learn that they can eat generous or even unlimited amounts of natural foods without gaining weight. The secret is that you must "fill up" on properly prepared lean meat, fish, chicken, eggs, skim milk, cottage cheese, salads, fruits, vegetables, juices, and whole grain products while *abstaining completely* from refined carbohydrates and greasy foods. (The diet of the average American is about 43 percent fat and includes more that 100 pounds of sugar a year!)

Note: If you enjoy an occasional cocktail, remember that alcohol contains more calories than any other food except fat.

EAT FIVE SMALL MEALS EACH DAY

Research has indicated that persons who eat five *small* meals daily rather than two or three large meals actually eat *less* and have less body fat as well as a lower level of blood cholesterol. It seems that frequent eating at regular intervals helps prevent overeating by keeping the appetite satisfied and the blood sugar at a normal, consistent level. Also, smaller meals do not contribute to an exaggerated appetite by stretching the stomach or overstimulating the pancreas. It's essential, however, that meals be made up entirely of natural foods. Even small amounts of refined foods can result in a pancreatic reaction that steals blood sugar and stores it as fat.

If you eat three meals a day, between-meal snacks of cottage cheese, fresh fruits, and raw vegetables will reduce mealtime appetite. Protein snacks are especially helpful in preventing the hunger, weakness, and low blood sugar that occurs in persons who are sensitive to the effects of carbohydrates.

If you do eat five small meals a day (or snack between meals), let your appetite mechanism guide you at mealtime. Eat only as much as you feel you need. Get up from the table when your appetite is satisfied and your stomach is comfortably full. Remember that the less you eat the better — as long as you eat a *variety* of natural foods.

Overloading your stomach will increase your heart rate and deprive your brain of adequate blood by diverting an excessive amount of blood to the digestive process. (This is why overeating makes you sleepy.) The pressure of an overloaded stomach against your diaphragm may also interfer with heart action. So even if you eat natural foods, you shouldn't stuff yourself. You should always quit eating *before* you feel that your stomach is completely full.

Reduce Slowly and Safely

The natural foods reducing diet is not a starvation diet. Diets that result in the loss of several pounds a week are dangerous. If your body burns more than two pounds of body fat a week, your diet may be deficient in essential food elements. The trick in reducing safely is to eliminate most of the fat in your diet and then cut down on your carbohydrates just enough to force your body to use some of its stored fat for energy. If carbohydrates are cut too drastically, an excessive amount of body fat will be burned for energy, resulting in a toxic condition caused by the by-products of fat metabolism.

On a low-fat natural foods diet, in which *all* processed foods are eliminated, a proper balance of protein, carbohydrate, and fat will automatically supply all the essential food elements and result in a gradual, progressive reduction of fat stores. Weight loss won't be as rapid as on a fad or crash diet but it will be permanent. Best of all, there'll be no starvation, and continued use of the diet will maintain an ideal bodyweight as well as build good health.

It isn't necessary to lose weight rapidly. If you lose only one pound a week, you can lose 52 pounds in a year! Diets that result in a loss of several pounds a week are impossible to follow for more than a few months at a time, either because they are deficient in essential food elements or because they are so unpalatable. When such diets are discontinued and old eating habits are resumed, empty fat cells are quickly filled and lost weight is rapidly regained.

If you eat properly, you can eat well, eat plenty, and never have to go on an unpleasant diet. With a diet properly balanced in natural foods, your bodyweight will automatically adjust itself and then remain at a healthy and desirable level. *Remember that a low-calorie diet that is rich in vitamins and minerals, with adequate amounts of protein, carbohydrate, and fat, is one of the secrets of longevity.*

Note: Many people on unbalanced "crash diets" take vitamin and mineral supplements to guard against nutritional deficiencies. It's important to remember, however, that natural foods may contain undiscovered vitamins, minerals, and enzymes that are essential for good health and a long life. For this reason, I do not recommend that anyone go on a diet that does not include some of all the basic natural foods. Even the indigestible cellulose supplied by fruits and vegetables is essential for good bowel health. If you want to supplement your diet with vitamins and minerals, you should do so *after* you have made sure that your diet is adequate.

How Wilmer T. Lowered His Blood Pressure by Reducing His Bodyweight

The case of Wilmer T. provides a good example of the health-building benefits of a natural foods reducing diet. Wilmer was only five feet, eight inches tall, but he weighed 225 pounds. His pulse rate was 90, with a blood pressure of 180 over 95 — abnormally high for a man only 36 years of age. His cholesterol and triglycerides were far above normal levels. After eating his meals, Wilmer had trouble breathing, and a burning pain in his chest pointed to possible ulcer or diaphragmatic hernia.

"I'm uncomfortable when I lie down," Wilmer complained, "and the slightest exertion makes me breathless. I don't feel well, and my love life has dropped to zero."

Poor Wilmer. Life was not pleasant for him, and his tendency to eat to console himself was cutting years off his life. Six months after he switched to a diet of natural foods, he had lost 40 pounds! His pulse rate and blood pressure were nearly normal, and his cholesterol and blood fat had dropped to a normal level. "I feel a hundred percent better," Wilmer reported. "And I'm getting plenty to eat."

Needless to say, I didn't have to encourage Wilmer to continue with his new eating habits. I know that when I see him six months from now, he won't be carrying around any excess body fat.

HOW YOUR MIND AND YOUR GLANDS CAN AFFECT YOUR WEIGHT

Persons who are unhappy or under stress will often eat to console themselves. In these cases, it's difficult or impossible to control food intake without first correcting underlying emotional problems. Some greatly obese persons are victims of an illness called the "night-eating syndrome," in which they eat little during the day and then consume large quantities of food during the night. Putting these people on a reducing diet may result in emotional stress that is more damaging to health than being overweight. If you are obese and eating seems to be a compulsion that relieves emotional stress, you should take whatever steps necessary to improve your state of mind before beginning a diet.

How to Control Your Bodyweight by Helping Your Thyroid

Most overweight is the result of overeating, but it can occasionally result from thyroid trouble. An iodine deficiency, for example, can result in a sluggish thyroid, which can lead to fatigue, overweight, and other symptoms.

Seafood is a good source of iodine. So be sure to eat seafood, preferably fish, at least once a week. Other nutrients are also essential for a healthy thyroid gland, and these must be supplied by the basic natural foods. You should not take pure iodine except when prescribed by a doctor. Excessive or improper use of iodine can be harmful and may even *cause* goiter.

Goiter, or enlargement of the thyroid gland, most commonly occurs at puberty or during pregnancy. Watch for any signs of swelling on the front of your neck.

If you live in the Rocky Mountains or in the Great Lakes area where the soil is deficient in iodine, you cannot depend upon vegetables for adequate iodine. Iodized salt can supply enough iodine to prevent the development of goiter. If you can't use salt for some reason, you should eat seafood at least once a week, or at least supplement your diet with kelp or some other product containing iodine.

When the thyroid is *underactive,* the metabolism slows down and the victim suffers from fatigue, constipation, dry and brittle hair, pale and puffy skin, sensitivity to cold, decreased perspiration, mental sluggishness, slow pulse, and overweight.

When the thyroid is *overactive,* the symptoms are just the opposite. The metabolism speeds up, causing nervousness, sweating, a rapid heart rate, weight loss, and an exaggerated appetite.

Whenever you suspect that you have thyroid trouble, you should always see a physician for an examination. Hyperthyroidism, for example, in which there is nervousness, inability to sleep, rapid weight loss, and protruding eyes, may be associated with a thyroid tumor.

BURN EXCESS CALORIES
BY STAYING ACTIVE

If you like to eat, you should stay physically active in order to burn excess calories. Such simple activities as walking, raking the yard, washing the car, or household chores can support a healthy appetite and prevent a build-up of body fat. If you take in more calories than you can use, you'll gain weight. It's as simple as that. If you have a weight problem, you must either eat less or exercise more — or both. If you eat natural foods, you can eat more without gaining weight and you won't have to take so much exercise to dispose of excess calories. Even if you aren't overweight, there are many good reasons why you should take regular exercise — to strengthen your heart as well as improve your physical appearance. There is now some evidence to indicate that regular exercise tunes body metabolism to dispose of excess calories 24 hours a day.

Recreational exercise, such as swimming, bicycle riding, rope jumping, tennis, or handball, will burn calories as effectively as calisthenics and other forms of exercise. It's very important that you enjoy the exercise you do if you plan to exercise regularly. Remember that it's better to stay active and eat well than to be inactive and starve yourself.

HOW TO GAIN WEIGHT
WITHOUT GETTING FAT

Persons who are underweight are likely to live longer than persons who are obese or overweight. If you are overly thin, however, you may have less resistance to infection and less reserve for recovery from illness. In many cases, bodyweight can be increased by eating more and exercising less. It's all right to increase your intake of natural carbohydrates supplied by fruits and vegetables, but you should never attempt to build up body fat by eating large amounts of fats and sweets. Too much fat can contribute to the development of cardiovascular disease, while too many sweets can damage the teeth or result in blood sugar problems.

Thiamine, or Vitamin B_1, might help you gain weight by stimulating your appetite and improving your digestion. If you feel that you have digestive problems, a supplement containing digestive enzymes might help. Make sure that the foods you eat are natural, tasty, and prepared and presented in an appetizing manner in order to stimulate your appetite.

If you fail to gain weight after several weeks of eating more and exercising less, see your doctor for a checkup. If you aren't suffering from disease or illness, or if you aren't *losing* weight, you shouldn't be overly concerned about being underweight. Some people are just naturally thin, making it difficult to gain weight. It's better to be thin than to be fat. So be careful not to add an excessive amount of body fat just so that you can weigh more. With most Americans living a sedentary life and eating large amounts of processed carbohydrates, being overweight is so common that few people ever complain about being underweight.

You can gain weight without adding fat by taking special exercises to increase the size of your muscles. Progressive resistance exercise with barbells and dumbbells offers the most effective and convenient way for both men and women to fill in bony areas with muscle tissue. If you're interested in such exercise, you can find a complete weight-training program in Chapter 1 of my book *Muscle Training for Athletes* (Parker Publishing Company).

HOW TO DELAY AGING WITH IMPROVED BODY MECHANICS

Take a look at yourself in the mirror. Do your shoulders slump? Is your upper back rounded? What about your abdomen? Is it disfigured by a pot belly?

If your body is not erect, flat, and properly aligned, your body mechanics may be a factor in the development of diseases and aches and pains that will surely shorten your life. Pressure on organs, blood vessels, and nerves, for example, can interfere with the function of important organs and cause a variety of symptoms. Strain on joints contributes to the development of arthritis, sore muscles, and other mechanical problems.

Vivian R. was only 38 years of age when she began to suffer from the signs and symptoms of "old age slump." She had burning pains in the muscles on her back. Shooting pains radiated around her ribs into her chest. Muscle soreness and headache plagued her constantly. Every morning around 3 a.m. she was awakened from sound sleep by soreness and stiffness in her thoracic spine. Vivian's symptoms had resulted from long hours slumping over a sewing machine. Even when she wasn't sewing, she slumped badly. Barbers, dentists, clerks, and other persons who work in a slumped or static posture for long hours each day often suffer from "old age slump." Muscles become inflamed from chronic tension. Spinal joints, inflamed by a postural strain, often ache after lying in bed for several hours. If the postural strains causing these symptoms are not relieved, permanent changes in the muscles and bones of the back can result in chronic symptoms that become progressively worse with aging.

All you have to do to reverse the aging influence of a slumping spine is to sit and stand correctly and take a simple exercise while lying down. Improving your posture will improve your body mechanics and make you feel better, look better, and work better. Vivian R., who followed the simple suggestions I've outlined for improving body mechanics, was able to relieve symptoms that had plagued her for several years. It's never too late to improve your body mechanics.

The role that posture and body mechanics play in the aging process is becoming increasingly more appreciated by physicians who specialize in geriatrics, or diseases of the aged. "Better postured individuals probably have fewer defects, enjoy better health, and live longer in good health than those with a seriously distorted skeleton," wrote Dr. Joseph Freeman, M.D., in the American Medical Association publication *Health Aspects of Aging.*

**How to Protect Your
Spine with Good Posture**

Good posture in a standing position can be maintained simply by "standing tall" so that your spine does not slump. Remember that as you grow older your vertebrae tend to become soft. If your upper back remains in an habitually slumped position, the softened vertebrae soon become compressed so that the slump becomes permanent. Then, as time passes, the pull of gravity creates a hump back or "dowager's hump" that aggravates arthritic aches and pains and makes you look much older than you really are. All this can be prevented by sitting and standing tall. Once good posture becomes a habit, you won't have to make a conscious effort to sit and stand correctly.

HOW TO LIE DOWN
AND STRAIGHTEN YOUR SPINE

If you're showing signs of a slump in your upper back, there's a simple exercise that you can do to forcefully straighten your spine.

Sofa-cushion pullover. Lie down on the floor (on your back) with a thick, hard cushion under your shoulder blades. Hold a light weight in both hands, at arm's length over your chest. Lower the weight back over your head with straight arms while inhaling deeply. This will correct the slump in your back by expanding your rib cage and extending your spine. Ten or 12 repetitions should be adequate. Be sure to lift your chest as high as you can in each repetition, while the weight is being lowered over your head to the floor. A ten-pound sandbag, or a brick in each hand, can be used as weights.

Carpet-roll spine straightener. If a shoulder problem does not permit you to do straight-arm pullovers, there's another way to forcibly extend your spine — and it can be done without any muscular effort whatsoever.

Roll up a large towel or a piece of carpet padding so that it forms a cylinder that's not over six inches thick. Place the cylinder across the middle of your upper back and lie on it relaxed for a few seconds a couple of times each day.

Note: Do not use the carpet-roll spine straightener if it causes pain or discomfort.

How to Stretch Out on a Slant Board

Lying on a slant board with your feet anchored at the high end of the board is a fine, effortless way to stretch out your spine and reverse the compression that gravity places on joints and organs. Lie relaxed on the board for several minutes. Select an elevation that feels most comfortable to you. (See Life Extender #4 for more information on how to use a slant board.)

If you have a sagging abdomen, do a few trunk curls while lying on the board. All you have to do is contract your abdominal muscles while curling your head and shoulders up from the board.

HOW TO TONE YOUR
BODY WITH A ROCKING CHAIR

When you sit in a chair, you should sit erect, all the way back in the chair, so that your spine won't slump. If you sit a great deal, you'd be better off sitting in a rocking chair. Using your muscles in a to-and-fro rocking motion will tone muscles, stimulate the circulation of blood, and help prevent clogging of blood vessels.

In order to make sure that your spine is properly supported and aligned while you sit, you can place a small pad in the small of your back. A pocket-size paperback book wrapped in a small hand towel will be adequate.

Don't sit too much each day, even if you sit in a rocking chair. Prolonged pressure against the back of your thighs and knees might interfere with the flow of arterial and venous blood in your legs, contributing to the development of varicose veins and blood clots. Walk as much as you can each day. If your job forces you to sit, use your rest breaks to walk in order to stimulate the circulation of blood.

BEWARE OF PROLONGED BED REST

When illness strikes and you are confined to home, don't stay in bed any more than necessary. Prolonged bed rest has many harmful effects on the body. A slowdown in circulation, for example, leads to stagnation of blood and the formation of clots. The heart grows weaker and pumps less blood. Fluids accumulate in the lungs and contribute to the development of pneumonia. Skeletal muscles shrink and become weak. Bones lose calcium and become brittle, and so on.

Remember that muscles must be *used* to maintain their usefulness and to aid the heart in the circulation of blood. Bones that are not placed under stress dump their calcium into the blood, contributing to the formation of kidney and bladder stones. Prolonged bed rest can also paralyze the bowels and clog the colon with a severe form of constipation. Your whole body suffers when it is forced to lie in bed day after day.

It isn't necessary to stay in bed to recover from such minor ailments as colds. Persons who go to bed unnecessarily may only delay their recovery and lower their resistance. If you are forced to go to bed with an acute or chronic illness, get out of bed whenever possible and walk around a little.

Movement is life. Keep your body youthful and healthy by staying active. Get the sleep you need, get adequate rest, and then get out of bed. Be guided by the way you feel. If you don't feel ill enough to stay in bed, chances are you'll get along better out of bed. There are few ailments or injuries that would force you to remain in bed 24 hours a day. Don't let your body waste away with inactivity or prolonged bed rest.

Summary

1. Obesity, or gross overweight, is a common cause of diseases that contribute to premature aging and death.
2. Simply eliminating sugar and white flour products from the diet would solve the overweight problem for most people.
3. A diet made up of a variety of fresh, low-fat natural foods, prepared without grease or oil, will automatically supply balanced amounts of vitamins, minerals, protein, carbohydrate, and fat.
4. Five small meals a day, rather than three large meals, may help reduce bodyweight by keeping the stomach small and the appetite satisfied.
5. A natural foods reducing diet may result in a loss of only a few pounds of fat a week, but the loss is per-

manent and the diet can be followed for a lifetime.

6. Regular physical activity will improve health as well as help control bodyweight.

7. Persons who are underweight should not attempt to gain weight by eating fats and sweets, since both contribute to the development of cardiovascular disease.

8. Sitting and standing tall will prolong your life by improving your body mechanics and preventing the development of disease.

9. A special exercise, a slant board, and a rocking chair can do wonders for your body mechanics and your circulation.

10. Prolonged bed rest weakens the body and contributes to premature aging, so don't stay in bed any longer than necessary in recovering from injury or illness.

LIFE EXTENDER #10

How to Put New
Bounce in Your Legs,
New Spring in Your Step

If you follow the instructions outlined in this book and take good care of yourself, chances are you'll live a long and healthy life. But what about your feet? In order to be as active as you should be to maintain a high level of fitness and to do all the things you desire to do, you'll have to depend upon your feet for exercise and transportation. So far, nothing has been said about the feet, and few doctors will look at your feet in checkup and examination procedures. What's more, most physicians know very little about the feet, and even less about treating them.

With Life Extender #10, you'll learn how to take care of your feet and legs, and how to use home remedies in the care of common foot ailments.

When your feet hurt, you hurt all over. And when your feet can't go, you can't go. With strong and healthy feet, you can benefit from tonics that put new bounce in your legs and new spring in your step. In addition to contributing to the look and feel of youth, a good pair of feet will contribute to the posture and the attitude you need to be successful in life. Without the hindrance and the distraction of painful, broken-down feet, you'll get more pleasure out of life, and you'll live longer.

HOW STELLA IMPROVED HER HEALTH BY HELPING HER FEET

Stella C. was only 36 years of age when her feet started to give her trouble. She had sharp pains in the front part of her feet when she walked. Bunions, corns, and calluses made it difficult to wear shoes. In addition to aching feet, Stella began to complain of backache and headache. She became more and more inactive, and spent more time sitting around the house. As a result, she gained weight. Her blood pressure and cholesterol started a dangerous climb. She felt bad and looked old.

Stella didn't know it, but *all* of her troubles stemmed from her feet! When she changed shoe styles and used some of the home remedies described in this chapter, her foot troubles began to disappear. She became more active and spent more time out of doors. The excess fat on her body slowly melted away. Her blood pressure dropped and her aches and pains disappeared as if by magic. Stella soon appeared to be getting younger rather than older!

If you have foot trouble of any type, your feet may be a factor in the development of many of your aging complaints. Even if you do not have any obvious foot trouble, you'll be well rewarded if you'll give your feet the attention they deserve.

HOW TO WEAR SHOES PROPERLY

Improperly fitted shoes can cripple your feet. Since you wear shoes for the greater part of each day, it's very important to make sure that the shoes you wear conform to the size and shape of your feet. Shoe heels should be as low as possible to prevent shortening of ankle tendons and tilting the pelvis. Women who insist on wearing high-heeled shoes should select working shoes with heels that are not over 1¼ inches high. The heels of dress shoes, which are to be worn for short periods of time only, should not be over two inches high.

Shoe heels that are too high can result in swayback and other postural disturbances. There may also be a tendency for the foot to slide forward in the shoe, jamming bones and pinching nerves. This can result in corns, calluses, bunions, arthritis, bursitis, nerve tumors, ingrowing toenails, and other painful and crippling foot disorders.

Persons who wear high-heeled shoes long enough will eventually be forced to abandon them because of foot trouble. Years of wearing high heels, however, shortens ankle tendons, making it difficult to switch suddenly from high heels to low heels without causing leg and back trouble.

If you must wear high heels, wear them only occasionally. The rest of the time, wear a good shoe that has a *low* heel. You can make sure that your ankle tendons don't shorten by doing the heel-lowering exercise described later in this chapter.

The toe of your shoes should be wide and blunt so that it won't squeeze your toes. Each shoe should be one-half to three-quarters of an inch longer than your longest toe. Be careful, however, not to get a shoe so long that the instep and arch portions do not fit your foot. If a shoe is properly fitted, it will feel comfortable and won't pinch your foot when you walk.

If you do not have fallen arches, you should not buy shoes that have built-in arch supports. You must *use* the muscles of your feet in order to keep your arches strong. Even a strong arch will become weak if it is constantly supported.

Strengthen Your Feet by Going Barefoot

Although you must wear shoes most of the time in a "civilized society," you should go barefoot every opportunity you get in order to strengthen the muscles supporting the 26 bones in each foot. Simple rubber sandals or "thongs" can be worn around the house and outdoors to protect the soles of your feet. If your feet are already broken down or very weak, however, you may not be able to go very long without the artificial support of a leather shoe. Persons with fallen arches may not be able to stand and walk normally without using arch supports to prevent painful leverage on the bridge of the foot. Remember that persons who are *born* with flat feet may be able to get along perfectly well without arch supports. So not everyone who has "flat feet" needs to wear arch supports.

Regardless of the apparent condition of your feet, you should not run and jump while barefoot if you are accustomed to wearing shoes. Weak feet must be strengthened in a slow and progressive manner before they can safely withstand a heavy load without support.

You'll learn later in this chapter how to strengthen your feet and how to care for broken-down feet. If your feet haven't been deformed by years of abuse and torture with "stylish shoes," you can regain full use of your feet with special exercises, home-treatment methods, and properly fitted shoes.

HOW TO STRENGTHEN YOUR ARCHES

The bony bridge forming the arch of your feet is very vulnerable to strain. When you walk, the arch of your foot acts as a lever to lift your bodyweight and propel you forward. Ligaments hold the bones of the arch together, but the foot depends upon muscles for support and mobility. If the muscles get weak, the ligaments become strained and the bones of the foot sag.

Walking barefoot in beach sand is a good exercise for the feet. Picking up marbles or a towel by grasping them with the toes is a popular and effective foot exercise. One of the best exercises, however, is simply rising up and down on your toes. This simple exercise strengthens the muscles that use the foot as a lever. In order to make sure that the exercise doesn't shorten your ankle tendons, you should do it with the front part of your feet supported by a thick board. Then, when you lower your heels to the floor, you'll get a stretch on your ankle tendons. Rise up and down on your toes for 12 or more times, until your calf muscles become fatigued. You may do this exercise while wearing shoes, preferably tennis shoes or some other soft, semi-supporting shoe.

GOOD FOOT POSTURE IS ALSO IMPORTANT

No matter what type of shoes you wear, how strong your feet are, or whether you wear shoes or not, you should always try to walk and stand with your toes pointed fairly straight ahead. And in order to make sure that your arches don't sag, you should consciously lift your arches a little so that most of your weight is supported on the outside edges of the soles of your feet. Such foot posture will protect your arches and balance your body mechanics so that there is no strain on your ankles, knees, hips, and lower back.

Bad foot posture can result in a variety of aches and pains that reach all the way from your feet to your neck. When the toes point too far outward, for example, the arches sag and the ankles roll inward, throwing the entire body out of balance. One of my patients, 54 year old Glen T., suffered constantly from arthritic pains in his spine. Nothing he did seemed to provide more than temporary relief. When steps were taken to correct an unsightly slew-footed stance, however, his symptoms were almost totally eased. He still had spinal arthritis, but taking the strain off his spine by improving his foot posture eliminated irritation of arthritic spurs.

In most cases, bad foot posture can be corrected with special exercises. In stubborn cases, heel and sole wedges prescribed by a podiatrist or an orthopedist may be needed to force correction of the feet.

For your health's sake as well as for a youthful step, it's essential that you practice good foot posture as well as wearing properly fitted shoes.

HOW TO IMPROVE YOUR
CIRCULATION TO SAVE YOUR FEET

As you grow older, chances are you'll suffer from some type of foot trouble, no matter how well you take care of your feet. Modern shoes and concrete walks place an abnormal strain on everyone's feet. Too much support along with inadequate exercise makes the feet weak and more susceptible to strain or injury. The bones of the feet tend to become brittle with age and are more easily fractured. Arthritis, poor circulation, diabetes, and other disorders also affect the feet. Some can be serious, resulting in disability or even *loss* of a foot.

Poor circulation probably poses the greatest danger to the feet. Your feet are a long way from your heart, and the uphill flow of venous blood (from your feet to your heart) is greatly hindered by the pull of gravity. Without regular walking exercises to stimulate blood flow, circulation in your feet and legs tends to slow down dangerously. Walk as much as you can. When you aren't walking, elevate your legs to drain venous blood out of your feet.

Atherosclerosis or hardened arteries is the greatest cause of poor circulation in the feet of persons past middle age. Hard fat accumulating in the arteries interferes with the circulation of blood. The dietary measures recommended under Life Extender #4 will help overcome the effects of hardened arteries. The nicotine from cigarette smoke can greatly complicate arteriosclerosis by constricting blood vessels. Even if you do not have hardened arteries, you should not smoke cigarettes if the circulation in your feet is poor.

Wading in cold water might trigger dangerous constriction of blood vessels in the feet. An attorney who spent a weekend wading in cold water on a duck-hunting trip noticed a few days later that all of the toes on one foot were purple in color. When he showed me his foot, I advised him to quit smoking and to see a physician immediately. Unfortunately, he delayed in seeking proper care and eventually had to have his toes amputated. He could have lost his foot and leg as well!

Try to avoid prolonged chilling of your feet on hunting, fishing, or camping trips. It isn't worth the risk.

Watch Out for Diabetes!

Diabetes can contribute to the development of hardened arteries, and it can greatly complicate circulatory problems in the feet. Infections, burns, and injuries around the feet and ankles are difficult to heal when the blood is loaded with sugar. You should, of course, try to *prevent* the development of diabetes by eliminating sugar and refined carbohydrates from your diet.

The older you become the more important it is to watch your diet. The reducing diet recommended under Life Extender #9 will help keep your blood sugar down. Don't wait until your doctor tells you that you have diabetes to begin thinking about prevention. Have your blood sugar tested at least once a year.

HOW TO FLUSH AWAY LEG CRAMPS

An advanced case of hardened arteries in your legs can certainly take the spring out of your step. Lack of an adequate supply of blood and oxygen to the muscles of the lower leg can make it difficult or impossible to walk more than a few minutes without leg ache and cramps. Turn back to Life Extender #4 and study the material on how to keep your arteries youthful for a longer life. You'll find some specific recommendations for "intermittent claudication," which is the name doctors give to leg cramps that occur while walking.

When leg cramps occur at night because of poor circulation or hardened arteries, it may be necessary to get out of bed and walk in order to stimulate the flow of blood. Thus, while too much walking might result in leg ache caused by an oxygen deficiency, inactivity can result in cramps caused by a slowdown in circulation.

An alcoholic drink will sometimes relieve the symptoms of hardened arteries by dilating the blood vessels. If walking around your bedroom does not relieve leg cramps that occur in the middle of the night, one or two ounces of whiskey or brandy might do the trick. Niacin or nicotinic acid, a B vitamin, might also improve circulation by dilating or widening blood vessels.

Note: Excessive use of alcohol may damage your liver. Large doses of niacin have been known to cause jaundice. So be careful not to go overboard with either of these remedies.

Many people who take niacin will experience a "hot flash" that causes the skin to become red, hot, and flushed with blood. This is a harmless reaction, but if it is severe or uncomfortable you should probably reduce your dosage of niacin to less than 50 milligrams — or switch to niacinamide.

HOW TO PREVENT
CRIPPLING BY VARICOSE VEINS

After middle age, varicose veins is a common crippler of the feet and legs. A weakness of the valves in the veins of the legs allows blood to back up in the veins until they are swollen and heavy with blood. The flow of venous blood slows to a trickle, causing stagnation that deprives the tissues of adequate oxygen and nutrients. This can result in aching, fatigue, cramps, swollen ankles, and discoloration in the feet and legs.

Elevating your legs will aid the flow of venous blood through your feet and legs. All you have to do is prop your feet up on your desk or lie on the floor and place your feet on a chair seat. Wrapping your lower leg from your foot to your knee with a wide (2- to 4-inch) elastic bandage will aid circulation by keeping varicose veins compressed. Begin the wrapping by taking a turn or two around your ankle and under your arch before beginning an overlapping spiral up your leg. Walking while your legs are wrapped will aid your leg muscles in pumping blood.

Special Care for
Phlebitis and Leg Ulcers

Varicose veins sometimes become inflamed and clogged, causing swelling, pain, and tenderness in the lower leg. When this happens, it may be necessary to go to bed and keep your legs elevated for several days. Mildly warm or cool compresses, whichever feel best, can be used to relieve pain and stimulate circulation. When the symptoms subside and you get back on your feet, elastic hose or an elastic bandage can be used to aid circulation and prevent swelling. A Vitamin E supplement will help prevent the formation of blood clots.

The treatment of varicose ulcers may also require rest in

bed, with daily applications of towels that have been wrung out in warm, salty water. Elevating the foot of the bed three or four inches will aid circulation.

If you're unable to treat a varicose ulcer with bed rest, you might be able to stay on your feet by wearing a "gelatin boot." This is a rigid wrapping of gauze and gelatin that will keep tissues and veins compressed so that circulation will be improved while walking.

How to Make a Gelatin Boot

Rub a little petrolatum or Vaseline over the ulcer and cover it with a sterile gauze dressing. Then wrap the leg from the foot to the knee with an overlapping layer of gauze. Make sure that the gauze isn't folded or wrinkled.

Melt a couple packages of plain gelatin in the top of a double boiler. Paint the gauze with a coat of warm, liquid gelatin. Wrap the leg with another layer of gauze and then paint on another coat of gelatin. Repeat this procedure three or four times, finishing with a heavy coat of gelatin. Leave the boot on for about six days.

When the boot is removed, wash the leg with soap and water and apply rubbing alcohol. If the ulcer hasn't healed, wait a couple of days before applying another boot.

An abbreviated ulcer wrapping. If you don't want to use a full gelatin boot, try this abbreviated wrapping: Cover the ulcer with Vaseline and gauze. Then cover the gauze with a sponge rubber pad that's about three-fourths of an inch thick and large enough to extend one inch beyond the margins of the ulcer. Over this, snugly wrap an elastic bandage that extends about two inches above and below the ulcer. Change the dressing once or twice a week for one to three weeks.

Note: Always see your doctor when a varicose ulcer develops. Leg ulcers are difficult to cure, and they heal slowly. Special cleaning procedures and medication may be needed to prevent infection.

HOW TO COPE WITH FOOT ARTHRITIS

Years of wear and tear and improper shoes can cause arthritis in the bones of the feet. Once arthritis does de-

velop, there is a certain amount of discomfort and disability
that may be permanent. So be sure to do all you can to *prevent* the development of arthritis in your feet. When the
symptoms of arthritis do begin to develop, there are many
home-treatment methods that may be helpful. When you have
any type of foot pain, however, you should be examined by a
podiatrist or an orthopedist to rule out more serious problems
before beginning home treatment. When foot pain results from
hardened arteries or inadequate blood flow, for example, hot
applications applied to the feet may cause tissue damage. You
should *never* apply heat to your feet when they are discolored
by a circulatory disorder. When in doubt, warm your feet with
woolen socks and blankets. A heating pad applied to your
abdomen will reflexly increase the flow of blood in your
feet.

Gout is a common cause of foot pain. A special diet (see
Life Extender #6) is sometimes effective in controlling gout,
but in severe cases it must be controlled with medication.
A simple blood test for uric acid can be used to diagnose
gout.

When the symptoms of foot arthritis begin after middle
age, they are usually the result of *osteoarthritis,* which can
be treated at home. Arthritis that begins before the age of
forty, however, may be *rheumatoid arthritis,* which may require specialized medical care to prevent crippling. Rheumatoid arthritis should always be suspected when the foot or
ankle is swollen.

Let a physician, preferably an orthopedist, diagnose your
foot pain. I once X-rayed the feet of a 70 year old man who
had been told by a number of doctors that his foot trouble
was being caused by arthritis. The X-ray revealed that one
of the bones in the arch of the crippled foot had completely
crumbled, leaving only a fragment where there should have
been a key supporting bone. Special care by an orthopedic
specialist could have prevented years of pain and disability.

When the bones of the feet become brittle because of
poor circulation, aging, or calcium deficiency, *fractures* may
occur spontaneously during such simple activities as walking.

"March fractures" commonly occur as a result of unaccustomed jogging.

Moist Heat Is Best
for Foot Arthritis

Once you feel confident that your foot problems are caused by simple arthritis, you may use hot water or *moist heat applications* to relieve symptoms. Immersing your feet in a pan of comfortably hot water, for example, may give blessed relief. The contrast bath described under Life Extender #6 will stimulate circulation and relieve symptoms as well as help strengthen bones. Supplementing your diet with bone meal tablets enriched with Vitamin D will keep your feet supplied with bone-building minerals.

Any of the heating techniques described under Life Extender #6 can be used to treat foot arthritis. It's probably more convenient and more effective, however, to immerse your feet in hot water. You may use the paraffin bath on your feet if you are careful not to get the wax too hot. Even if you have good circulation, you should be careful not to burn your feet.

Calcium Doesn't Cause Bone Spurs

Many people who have arthritis with "calcium deposits" feel that taking calcium will only aggravate their condition. Actually, the calcium in *arthritic spurs* builds up in response to chronic bony irritation. The amount of calcium in the diet has nothing to do with the formation of these spurs. If the diet is deficient in calcium, an arthritic process will take calcium from the bones to form spurs. Increasing the amount of calcium in the diet will *not* contribute to the development of arthritic spurs. You must have calcium in your diet to keep your bones from becoming soft or brittle. So don't hesitate to supplement your diet with bone meal just because you have arthritis or "calcium deposits."

HOW TO DEAL WITH
FOOT-CRIPPLING BUNIONS

Just about every woman who wears high-heeled shoes with pointed toes will eventually develop a bunion. The downhill slant of the shoe forces the foot to slide forward, jamming the toes into the pointed section of the shoe. This bends the big toe inward and places pressure on the outer margin of the toe. As a result, the big toe literally dislocates, and a build-up of bone and bursa at the base of the toe forms a painful enlargement. Once a bunion forms, it's difficult to wear a leather shoe. The slightest pressure against the bunion causes a recurrence of swelling and pain. It's sometimes necessary to slit a shoe in order to relieve pressure on a bunion.

Prevention is the best treatment for bunions. It's essential to fit shoes so that they don't squeeze your toes. If you must wear tapered shoes that press your big toe inward a little, pull the shoes off every chance you get and stretch your big toe by pulling it forward and away from the other toes. A pad of lamb's wool placed between the big toe and the first toe will help hold the big toe in a corrected position.

HOW TO GET RID OF CORNS AND CALLUSES

Corns and calluses on the feet are almost always caused by improperly fitted shoes. In most cases, all you have to do to get rid of a corn or callus is to relieve it of pressure or irritation. This means changing shoe style or shoe size. You can speed the disappearance of corns and calluses by protecting them with special pads and by filing them or rubbing them with pumice.

You can purchase "corn pads" in any drug store — or you can make your own. Just cut a hole in a piece of felt and fit it over a painful corn.

Calluses that develop on the bottom of the feet can be caused by bad foot posture as well as by improperly fitted shoes. So be sure to observe the rules of good foot posture, as outlined earlier in this chapter.

Corns and calluses that have been softened by soaking the feet in hot, soapy water can be trimmed with a *dull,* used razor blade that has been sterilized by alcohol. To make sure that you don't cut too deeply, cut away only a small portion of the corn with the razor blade and then use an emery board to finish the job. Always wash your feet before trimming a corn, and always stop cutting or filing if blood appears. Avoid cutting whenever possible. It's safer to use an emery board.

Regular use of an emery board will keep a corn from building back up. Remember, however, that disappearance of a corn will depend primarily upon properly fitted shoes. As long as pressure or irritation is present, a corn or callus will keep recurring.

When corns develop between the toes, a little Vaseline or lamb's wool between the affected toes will reduce friction and relieve irritation.

Note: If you have diabetes, hardened arteries, or poor circulation in your feet, let a podiatrist trim your corns and calluses in order to avoid risk of infection.

HOW TO RELIEVE FOOT
PAIN WITH A METATARSAL PAD

When the front portion of the foot is painful during walking or standing, a metatarsal pad taped to the bottom of the foot may relieve the pain. Normally, the small, oval pad would be placed under the front of the foot, just behind the painful area. This will shift the weight off the painful area and relieve pressure on jammed joints and pinched nerves. Most shoe stores sell these pads, and most shoe salesmen can show you how to use them.

WHAT TO DO ABOUT HEEL SPURS

A heel spur is a sharp, bony growth on the bottom of the heel bone. It doesn't always cause trouble, but when it does it makes walking difficult and painful.

The first thing you should do to relieve the symptoms of a heel spur is to wear shoes with rubber heels. This may cushion the heel enough to prevent painful pressure on the spur. If that doesn't help, try placing a sponge rubber pad inside your shoe under the painful heel. An arch support may lift the foot enough to relieve pressure on a painful heel. A piece of felt or rubber with a hole cut in it, placed in your shoe so that the hole is centered over the painful spot, is often effective in relieving painful pressure. If nothing else helps, it may be necessary to gouge a hole into the shoe heel (from the inside) and then fill the cavity with sponge rubber.

HOW TO REJUVENATE YOUR FEET

The feet must withstand a great amount of abuse and strain. Yet, they are the most neglected part of the body. You can give your feet a treat, and improve your health, with special treatment applied at home.

An occasional *contrast bath* will stimulate circulation and open blood vessels in the feet. Immerse your feet in comfortably hot water for three minutes and then in comfortably cold water for one minute. Repeat the procedure at least twice, ending with hot water. Dry your feet thoroughly. Then apply a little vegetable oil to your feet and massage them with your hands. Wipe the oil from your feet with a *dry* wash cloth. This will leave just enough oil on the skin to be beneficial.

If you have corns between your toes, cover them with a little Vaseline before putting your socks and shoes on.

A FEW ADDITIONAL HINTS ON FOOT CARE

Always dry your feet thoroughly after each bath, especially between your toes. Then powder your toes with a good medicated powder. This will help prevent the growth of fungus that causes athlete's foot.

Wear thick cotton socks, preferably white. Nylon socks do not absorb moisture and will encourage the growth of fungus. You should not wear stretch socks, since they tend to squeeze the toes and cause ingrowing toenails.

Lamb's wool placed between the toes will relieve irritation that leads to the development of corns. You should never put cotton between your toes, since cotton tends to collect and hold moisture.

Always trim toenails straight across and then file off the sharp corners (to prevent snagging of hose). When nails are cut too far down on each side, they tend to grow into the flesh. In many cases, ingrown toenails are caused by tight shoes and stretch socks that *press* the nail into the flesh.

HOW TO PEP UP YOUR STEP WITH TONICS

If your feet are in good shape but you are "too tired" to use them, you may need a "tonic" to perk you up. A simple cold water shower will provide you with a surge of energy. The B vitamins are often recommended as a source of power for the nervous system. Rather than take thiamine hydrochloride (synthetic Vitamin B_1) or an injection of Vitamin B_{12}, it might be best to take *all* the B vitamins in a "B complex" formula. You can purchase "high potency Vitamin B complex" in any drug store or health food store. Brewer's yeast and desiccated liver are good sources of all the B vitamins. I usually recommend both of them for "tired" middle-aged and elderly persons.

If you happen to be deficient in iron, foods rich in iron will relieve fatigue and restore energy. Liver is one of the best sources of iron, and it's rich in Vitamin B_{12}. Wheat germ is also a good source of iron and B vitamins.

With good feet and plenty of energy, you'll have a better chance of *enjoying* a long, healthy life.

Summary

1. In addition to causing pain and crippling disability, the inactivity resulting from bad feet can contribute to poor health and premature aging.
2. Properly fitted shoes are essential in the treatment and prevention of corns, calluses, bunions, ingrown toenails, and other common foot ailments.
3. Healthy arches should not be supported, and the muscles of the feet should be strengthened by going barefoot and by doing special exercises.
4. Good foot posture protects the feet and relieves strain on the ankles, legs, knees, hips, and lower back.
5. Poor circulation in the feet, complicated by hardened arteries, diabetes, cigarette smoking, and nutritional deficiencies, can cause serious disability if corrective measures aren't taken.

6. Varicose veins in the legs can lead to phlebitis, leg ulcers, and other problems if they are not controlled with self-help methods.

7. The home remedies described in this chapter can relieve the pain and disability caused by foot arthritis, gout, bunions, corns, calluses, and heel spurs.

8. Special pads may be used with properly fitted shoes to relieve jamming of bones and pinching of nerves in the foot.

9. Treating your feet with a contrast bath and then massaging them with vegetable oil will literally rejuvenate your feet.

10. Brewer's yeast, desiccated liver, wheat germ, and other foods rich in iron and B vitamins will boost your energy and put new spring in your step.

CONCLUSION

Although many of the life extenders recommended in this book will provide immediate relief from suffering, you should not expect to become youthful overnight. Remember that any longevity program must be followed over a long period of time if it is to be effective. Such a program should, in fact, become a part of your way of life, so that everything you do throughout the day — every day — will contribute to better health and a longer life. This is not difficult to do. It's simply a matter of replacing bad habits with good habits.

Once you acquire good living habits, life is much easier and more pleasant. Best of all, as the months and years go by, you can be confident that your health will improve and the aging process will be delayed. In many cases, the aging process may actually *reverse* itself.

There is no more important investment than a little time and effort to improve your health and lengthen your life. This book tells you what to do and how to do it. Keep it handy for daily use and constant reference.

INDEX

Y

Yeast, brewer's, 32-33
Yogurt:
    aids assimilation and absorption, 30
    bacteria, 30
    benefits of milk, 31
    colon, 30
    commercial starter, 31
    development, 31
    intestinal health, 30-31
    make at home, 31

Yogurt: (*cont.*)
    mild or acid, 31
    milk allergy, 167
    natural antibiotic, 30
    orally taken drugs and antibiotics, 30
    quality, 31
    stomach ulcer, 174
    used in enemas, 30
    varieties, 30
    Vitamin K and certain B vitamins, 30
    with other foods, 31